Atlas of Developmental Anomalies in Experimental Animals
実験動物発生異常アトラス

Visceral Anomalies
内臓異常

Edited by Project of the Terminology Committee of the Japanese Teratology Society

日本先天異常学会用語委員会　編集

FOREWORD

The first harmonized terminology (Version 1) of developmental anomalies in experimental animals, which was developed by members of the International Federation of Teratology Societies including North America, Europe and Japan, was published in 1997 (Teratology, 55:249-292, 1997; Cong. Anom., 37:165-210,1997). The Japanese version of this terminology was published the following year (Cong. Anom., 38:153-237, 1998).

The revised edition (Version 2) of this terminology was published by society members in 2009 (Cong. Anom., 49(3):123-246, 2009; Birth Defects Research (Part B), 86:227-327, 2009; Repro. Toxicol., 28:371-434, 2009). This version utilizes simple descriptions and is useful for laboratory technicians.

The Terminology Committee of the Japanese Teratology Society established "A Database of Congenital Anomalies in Laboratory Animals" in the society homepage in 2010 and provided photographs of malformations and variations submitted by many Japanese companies. Submitted photographs were reviewed by a terminology project, some members in the committee, and were registered in the database mentioned above.

This textbook, "Atlas of Congenital Anomalies in Experimental Animals", compiled photographs of visceral anomalies and variations with their associated explanations. We expect this to be used by researchers that conduct teratological studies and who review data of reproductive and developmental toxicity.

Table 1 shows list of visceral anomalies and variations based on the harmonized terminology (Version 2, 2009). However, organs/tissues and findings that could not be observed or confirmed/diagnosed in fetuses of mice, rats and rabbits were eliminated from the terminology list.

Table 2 shows harmonized findings of the atlas by the International Federation of Teratology Societies, compared with those in Mouse Phenotype (MP) ontology (Smith CL et al., 2005) and Human Phenotype (HP) ontology (Kohler S et al., 2014). This comparative list is meant to support researchers using transgenic animals or who encounter phenotypic abnormalities in human disease.

Smith CL et al. The Mammalian Phenotype Ontology as a tool for annotating, analyzing and comparing phenotypic information. Genome Biol. 6(1): R7, 2005
Kohler S et al. The Human Phenotype Ontology project: linking molecular biology and disease through phenotype data. Nucleic Acids Res. 42:D966, 2014

はじめに

　1960年代のサリドマイド薬禍を契機として、化合物の暴露による先天異常発現が問題となり、多くの研究者により実験動物を用いた発生毒性研究が進められました。また、これら研究成果の科学的信憑性を担保するため、催奇形性試験や生殖発生毒性試験に関するガイドラインも各国の規制当局により制定・改訂され、今日に至っています。しかし、実験動物を用いた試験・研究においては、実際に観察する発生異常の診断は、臨床で用いられている先天異常用語を参考にして行っていたのが現状でした。1997年に日欧米三極の研究者により実験動物での発生用語の統一が図られ、実験動物発生異常用語集 Version 1（Teratology, 55:249-292, 1997; Cong. Anom., 37:165-210,1997）が提示されました。また、翌年には日本語版として、「実験動物発生異常用語集」（Cong. Anom., 38:153-237, 1998）も発表されました。この用語集で用いられている所見名はいわゆる診断用語であり、試験・研究の実務担当者には扱いにくい面もあることから、より簡易な用語を用いた用語集 Version 2 として2009年に改訂されました（Cong. Anom., 49(3):123-246, 2009; Birth Defects Research (Part B), 86:227-327, 2009; Repro. Toxicol., 28:371-434, 2009）。

　これを受けて、日本先天異常学会 用語委員会は2010年、学会ホームページに「実験動物先天異常データベース」を開設し、Version 2 に規定された用語集の日本語版を掲載すると共に、それらに該当する写真の公開を行っています。これまで多くの企業、施設のご協力により、貴重な異常・変異の写真を提供していただきました。この場を借り、お礼申し上げます。委員会では、審査プロジェクトを組み、メンバーにより写真及びその診断、説明の妥当性を審査し、上記データベースに登録してきました。

　本アトラスは、生殖発生毒性研究を実施される研究者や生殖発生毒性を評価される方々に活用いただける様、上記データベースを基に実験動物の内臓異常及び変異の写真並びにその説明をまとめたものです。外表異常（Atlas of Developmental Anomalies in Experimental Animals – External Anomalies, 2015）に続き、本アトラスを出版します。

　Table 1 に所見名の一覧及び掲載された写真の番号を記載しました。所見の一覧については、上述の実験動物発生異常用語集 Version 2 (Cong. Anom., 49(3):123-246, 2009; Birth Defects Research (Part B), 86:227-327, 2009; Repro. Toxicol., 28:371-434, 2009)を基本として、和文も付加してあります。ただ、胎児では観察できない、あるいは、診断できない器官・組織や所見を除いて掲載してあります。

　また、近年、遺伝子解析技術の飛躍的な発展によって、先天異常学分野全般の研究が加速しています。今後、遺伝子改変動物の表現型の解析を通じた、遺伝子機能の決定、遺伝子変異とヒト遺伝性疾患の患者の症状の関係の研究の一層の展開が期待されます。遺伝子変異データがデジタルデータであるのに対して、表現型のデータはフォーマットの一定しないデータと見なされてきましたが、表現型をデジタル化可能な

コードとして国際標準化しようとする動きが進んでいます。著者らはこの動きに呼応するかたちで、本アトラスに示される表現型に対してコード (マウス、Mouse phenotype: Smith CL et al. The Mammalian Phenotype Ontology as a tool for annotating, analyzing and comparing phenotypic information. Genome Biol. 6(1): R7, 2005、及び、ヒト、Human phenotype: Kohler S et al. The Human Phenotype Ontology project: linking molecular biology and disease through phenotype data. Nucleic Acids Res. 42:D966, 2014) を示しました（Table 2 参照）。本アトラスが動物の胎児への薬物毒性の研究者のみならず、広く遺伝子改変動物やヒト遺伝性疾患の研究者にとって有用なレファレンスになればと願っています。

協力企業・施設

アステラス製薬株式会社
株式会社サンプラネット
住友化学株式会社
株式会社 LSI メディエンス
武田薬品工業株式会社

株式会社ボゾリサーチセンター
大日本住友製薬株式会社
大鵬薬品工業株式会社
財団法人残留農薬研究所

Project members of the Terminology Committee in Japanese Teratology Society

Yojiro Ooshima

Michio Fujiwara (Astellas Pharma Inc.)

Kazuhiro Chihara (Sumitomo Dainippon Pharma Co., Ltd.)

Yuko Izumi (Takeda Pharmaceutical Company Ltd.)

Yoshihiro Katsumata (BoZo Research Center Inc.)

Hiroshi Sumida (Hiroshima International University)

Makoto Ema (AIST)

Kenjiro Kosaki (Keio University)

Advisors

Kohei Shiota (Shiga University of Medical Science)

Stewart Jacobson (SNBL USA)

CONTENTS

Foreword

Table 1 List of Visceral Anomalies ··· 1

Table 2 Comparative List of This Atlas Findings, Mouse Phenotype, and Human Phenotype ···· 33

Photographs of Normal Fetuses in Rats ·· 37

Photographs of Visceral Anomalies

   1. General ·· 43

   2. Brain ·· 47

   3. Eye and Nose ·· 55

   4. Thoracic Organs ·· 67

   5. Heart ··· 81

   6. Vessel ·· 93

   7. Abdominal Organs ··· 139

   8. Reproductive Organs ··· 167

Table 1. List of Visceral Anomalies

Region / Organ / Structure	Observation		Synonym or Related Term	Ver. 1 Code No.	Definition	Note	Photo No.
General 全身	Abdomen 腹部	Cyst 嚢胞		New			
General 全身	Abdominal wall 腹壁	Cyst 嚢胞		New		Location and size should be defined 位置と大きさを特定する	
		Thin 菲薄		New		May be generalized or localized 全体あるいは局所の場合がある	
General 全身	Aneurysm 血管瘤			10125	Localized sac formed by dilatation of an artery or vein that is filled with blood 動脈あるいは静脈が拡張して形成された局所性の嚢で，血液を充満する		
General 全身	Situs inversus 内臓逆位	Abdominal 腹部		New	Mirror-image transposition of the abdominal viscera 腹部器官の位置が，正常に対して鏡像的		
		Thoracic 胸部		New	Mirror-image transposition of the thoracic viscera 胸部器官の位置が，正常に対して鏡像的		
		Total 胸腹部		10127	Mirror-image transposition of the abdominal and thoracic viscera 腹部と胸部器官の位置が，正常に対して鏡像的		1-1
General 全身	Thoracic wall 胸壁	Cyst 嚢胞		New		Location and size should be defined 位置と大きさを特定する	
Brain 脳	Brain 脳	Hole 嚢胞	Cyst	New	Appears as discrete 'hole' in fixed brain tissue 固定された脳では，孤在する穴のように見える	May be due to processing artifact アーティファクトによる場合がある	

Table 1. List of Visceral Anomalies

Region / Organ / Structure	Observation		Synonym or Related Term	Ver. 1 Code No.	Definition	Note	Photo No.
Brain 脳	Brain 脳	Large 大型(化)		New			
		Misshapen 形態異常		New		.	2-1
		Small 小型(化)		New			
Brain 脳	Cerebellum 小脳	Discolored 変色		New		May be generalized or localized 全体あるいは局所の場合がある	
		Large 大型(化)		New			
		Misshapen 形態異常		10132			
		Small 小型(化)		10134			
Brain 脳	Cerebrum 大脳	Discolored 変色		New		May be generalized or localized 全体あるいは局所の場合がある	
		Large 大型(化)		New			
		Misshapen 形態異常		10133			2-2
		Small 小型(化)		10135			
Brain 脳	Fourth ventricle 第四脳室	Dilated 拡張(化)	*Internal* hydrocephaly (10131), *Large fourth ventricle* *内水頭(症) (10131)*, 第四脳室大型(化)	New		See also Ventricles, dilated 「脳室，拡張」を参照	
Brain 脳	Lateral ventricle 側脳室	Dilated 拡張(化)	Dilated cerebral ventricle, *Internal hydrocephaly (10131)*, Large lateral ventricle 脳室拡張，*内水頭(症) (10131)*, 側脳室大型(化)	10128		Involvement of anterior portion of lateral ventricle, within olfactory lobe, may also be noted See also Ventricles, dilated 嗅葉に含まれる側脳室前方部分の障害が見られる場合がある 「脳室，拡張」を参照	2-3
Brain 脳	Olfactory lobe 嗅葉	Absent 欠損		New		To be used when laterality of absent lobe cannot be determined 欠損した葉の側性が決定できないときに使用する	

Table 1. List of Visceral Anomalies

Region / Organ / Structure	Observation		Synonym or Related Term	Ver. 1 Code No.	Definition	Note	Photo No.
Brain 脳	Olfactory lobe 嗅葉	Large 大型(化)		New			
		Single 単		New			
		Small 小型(化)		New			
Brain 脳	Perimeningeal space 髄膜周辺腔	Large 拡張(化)	*External hydrocephaly (10131)* 外水頭(症) (10131)	New	Increase in space between brain and skull 脳と頭蓋骨の間の空隙の増大	May be due to processing artifact アーティファクトによる場合がある	2-4
Brain 脳	Third ventricle 第三脳室	Dilated 拡張(化)	*Internal hydrocephaly (10131),* Large third ventricle 内水頭(症) (10131)、第三脳室大型(化)	New		See also Ventricles, dilated 「脳室，拡張」を参照	2-5
Brain 脳	Ventricles 脳室	Dilated 拡張(化)	*Internal hydrocephaly (10131),* Large ventricles 内水頭(症) (10131)、脳室大型(化)	New		See also separate observations for dilated lateral, third, and fourth ventricles. 側脳室，第三脳室および第四脳室の拡張に分けてもよい	
Ear 耳	Inner ear 内耳	Malpositioned 位置異常		New			
		Misshapen 形態異常		10136			
		Small 小型(化)		New			
Ear 耳	Inner/middle ear 内/中耳	Malpositioned 位置異常		New			
		Misshapen 形態異常		New			
		Small 小型(化)		New			
Ear 耳	Middle ear 中耳	Malpositioned 位置異常		New			
		Misshapen 形態異常		New			
		Small 小型(化)		New			

Table 1. List of Visceral Anomalies

Region / Organ / Structure	Observation		Synonym or *Related Term*	Ver. 1 Code No.	Definition	Note	Photo No.
Eye 眼	Aqueous chamber / humor 眼房/房水	Absent 欠損		New			
		Large 大型(化)		New			
		Small 小型(化)		New			
Eye 眼	Eye 眼	Absent 欠損	Anophthalmia 無眼球(症)	10137			3-1
		Large 大型(化)	Macrophthalmia, Megalophthalmia (-mus, -mos) 巨眼球(症)	10141	Large eye, eyeball 大きな眼、眼球		
		Malpositioned 位置異常		10142			
		Small 小型(化)	Microphthalmia 小眼球(症)	10143	Small eye, eyeball, globe of eye 小さい眼、眼球		3-2
Eye 眼	Lens 水晶体	Absent 欠損	Aphakia 無水晶体(症)	10138			
		Adhered to cornea 角膜に癒着		New			
		Altered texture 組織変化		New		Usually seen on cut surface of sectioned lens; May be generalized or localized 通常水晶体断面の表面に見られる；全体あるいは局所の場合がある	
		Double 重複	Duplicated 重複	New			
		Large 大型(化)		New			
		Misshapen 形態異常		10144			3-3

Table 1. List of Visceral Anomalies

Region / Organ / Structure	Observation		Synonym or *Related Term*	Ver. 1 Code No.	Definition	Note	Photo No.
Eye 眼	Lens 水晶体	Opacity 混濁	Cataract, Eye internal opacity 白内障、眼内部混濁	10139	Opacity of the crystalline lens 水晶体の混濁	If seen at fresh examination, deep in the eye, may be called 'internal opacity' since location cannot be definitive 新鮮臓器解剖の場合、局在が明確ではないため、「内部混濁」としてもよい May be artifact アーティファクトの場合がある	3-4
		Small 小型(化)		10147			
Eye 眼	Retina 網膜	Fold 皺襞		10146	Undulation of retinal layers 波状の網膜層	Characterization of severity is important 重篤度を示すことは重要である May be due to processing artifact アーティファクトによる場合がある	3-5
Eye 眼	Vitreous chamber / humor (body) 硝子体腔/液(体)	Absent 欠損		New			
		Large 拡張(化)		New			
		Small 小型(化)		New			
Naso-pharyngeal tract 鼻咽頭管	Nasal cavity 鼻腔	Large 大型(化)		10150			3-6
		Misshapen 形態異常		New			
		Small 小型(化)		10153			3-7
Naso-pharyngeal tract 鼻咽頭管	Nasal conchae 鼻甲介	Absent 欠損		10148			
		Fused 癒合		New			
		Large 大型(化)		New			
		Malpositioned 位置異常		10151			
		Misshapen 形態異常		New		Includes reduced number of convolutions 渦巻の数が少ないものも含まれる	
		Small 小型(化)		10154			

Table 1. List of Visceral Anomalies

Region / Organ / Structure	Observation		Synonym or *Related Term*	Ver. 1 Code No.	Definition	Note	Photo No.
Naso-pharyngeal tract 鼻咽頭管	Nasal septum 鼻中隔	Absent 欠損		10149			**3-8**
		Malpositioned 位置異常		10152			
		Misshapen 形態異常	Bent 屈曲	New			
		Not fused with palate 口蓋との癒合不全		New			
		Small 小型(化)		10155			
Thyroid gland 甲状腺	Thyroid gland 甲状腺	Absent 欠損		10156			
		Large 大型(化)		New			
		Malpositioned 位置異常		10157			
		Misshapen 形態異常		New			
		Small 小型(化)		New			
		Supernumerary lobe 分葉過剰	*Pyramidal lobe* *錐体葉*	New			
Thymus 胸腺	Thymic cord 胸腺索		Extra thymic tissue, Thymic remnant in the neck, Thymus long cranial 胸腺組織過剰、胸腺頸部残留、胸腺が頭蓋方向に長い	New	Partially undescended horn of thymus 部分的な胸腺の下降不全		**4-1**
Thymus 胸腺	Thymus 胸腺	Absent 欠損	Athymia, Athymism 無胸腺(症)	10158			
		Discolored 変色		New		May be generalized or localized 全体あるいは局所の場合がある	
		Fragmented 断片(化)		New	Multiple small fragments 多数の小さな断片		

Table 1. List of Visceral Anomalies

Region / Organ / Structure	Observation		Synonym or *Related Term*	Ver. 1 Code No.	Definition	Note	Photo No.
Thymus 胸腺	Thymus 胸腺	Large 大型(化)		New			
		Malpositioned 位置異常		10160			
		Misshapen 形態異常		10161			4-2
		Small 小型(化)		10162	Reduced size or remnant of thymus 小型、胸腺の痕跡		4-3
		Split 分離		10163			
		Supernumerary 過剰		10164			
Heart 心臓	Aortic valve 大動脈弁	Absent 欠損		10165			
		Large 大型(化)		10177			
		Misshapen 形態異常		10189		Includes alterations in number of cusps 心臓弁膜尖の数の異常を含む	
		Small 小型(化)		10195			
Heart 心臓	Atrial septum 心房中隔	Defect 欠損		10171	Postnatal communication between atria; includes defects of septa primum and secundum 心房間が生後も連絡した状態；一次中隔と二次中隔の欠損を含む	Not to be confused with the foramen ovale which normally remains open until birth 出生まで通常開存している卵円孔と混同しない	5-1
Heart 心臓	Atrium 心房	Malpositioned 位置異常		New			
		Misshapen 形態異常		New			
		Large 大型(化)	*Distended* *拡張(化)*	New			
		Small 小型(化)	*With no blood inside* *心房内に血液なし*	New			

Table 1. List of Visceral Anomalies

Region / Organ / Structure	Observation		Synonym or *Related Term*	Ver. 1 Code No.	Definition	Note	Photo No.
Heart 心臓	A-V canal 共通房室口(管) A-V = atrioventricular、房室	Persistent 遺残		10194	Defects of endocardial cushions resulting in low atrial and high ventricular septal defects 心内膜クッションの欠損による心房中隔下部と心室中隔上部の欠損		5-2
Heart 心臓	A-V ostium 房室口	Dilated 拡張(化)		20179	Enlargement of an atrioventricular orifice 房室口の拡大		
Heart 心臓	A-V septum 房室中隔	Defect 欠損		10175	Inappropriate communication between atrium and ventricle 心房と心室間の異常な連絡		
Heart 心臓	Foramen ovale 卵円孔	Premature closure 早期閉鎖		New		Foramen ovale is normally open in fetuses 卵円孔は胎児では通常開存している	5-3
Heart 心臓	Heart 心臓	Absent 欠損	Acardia 無心(症)	New			
		Large 大型(化)	Cardiomegaly 巨心(症)	10172			
		Malpositioned 位置異常	*Dextrocardia (right-sided heart)* 右胸心(右心)	10186		Levocardia (left-sided heart) is abnormal only in situs inversus; right-sided heart, previous code # 10176 左胸心(左心)の異常は逆位の場合のみ；右心、旧コード番号10176	
		Misshapen 形態異常		New			5-4
		Small 小型(化)	Microcardia 小心(症)	10188			
		Three-chambered 三腔	Cor triloculare 三腔心	10174	Three-chambered heart with two atria and a ventricle or one atrium and two ventricles 3つの腔(2つの心房と1つの心室あるいは1つの心房と2つの心室)のある心臓		

Table 1. List of Visceral Anomalies

Region / Organ / Structure	Observation		Synonym or Related Term	Ver. 1 Code No.	Definition	Note	Photo No.
Heart 心臓	Heart 心臓	Two-chambered 二腔	Cor biloculare 二腔心	10173	Two-chambered heart with an atrium and a ventricle 2つの腔(1つの心房と1つの心室)のある心臓		
Heart 心臓	Left A-V valve 左房室弁 A-V = atrioventricular; also known as bicuspid/mitral、房室；二尖弁/僧帽弁としても知られている	Absent 欠損		10167			
		Large 大型(化)		10180			
		Misshapen 形態異常		10190			5-5
		Small 小型(化)		10196			
Heart 心臓	Pulmonary valve 肺動脈弁	Absent 欠損		10169			
		Large 大型(化)		10181			
		Misshapen 形態異常		10191			Includes alterations in number of cusps 心臓弁膜尖の数の異常を含む	5-6
		Small 小型(化)		10197			
Heart 心臓	Right A-V valve 右房室弁 A-V = atrioventricular; also known as tricuspid、房室；三尖弁としても知られている	Absent 欠損		10170			
		Large 大型(化)		10182			
		Misshapen 形態異常		10192			Includes alterations in number of cusps. 心臓弁膜尖の数の異常を含む
		Small 小型(化)		10198			
Heart 心臓	Ventricle 心室	Double outlet 両大血管起始		New	Pulmonary trunk and aorta arise from same ventricle 肺動脈幹と大動脈が同じ心室から起始している	Usually associated with right ventricle 通常、右心室	5-7

Table 1. List of Visceral Anomalies

Region / Organ / Structure	Observation		Synonym or *Related Term*	Ver. 1 Code No.	Definition	Note	Photo No.
Heart 心臓	Ventricle 心室	Large 大型(化)		New		See Ventricular chamber and Ventricular wall; only to be used when heart has not been cut for examination 「心室腔」と「心室壁」項を参照；心臓を内部検査(切断)していない時のみに使用する	
		Small 小型(化)		New		See Ventricular chamber and Ventricular wall; only to be used when heart has not been cut for examination 「心室腔」と「心室壁」項を参照；心臓を内部検査(切断)していない時のみに使用する	
Heart 心臓	Ventricular chamber 心室腔	Large 拡張(化)		10183			
		Small 狭小(化)		10199			
Heart 心臓	Ventricular septum 心室中隔	Defect 欠損	*Incomplete VS, Membranous VSD, Muscular VSD, Perimembranous VSD* 心室中隔不完全、心室中隔膜性部欠損、心室中隔筋性部欠損，心室中隔膜周辺部欠損	New	An opening in the membranous and/or muscular septum between the ventricles 心室中隔の膜性部あるいは筋性部の孔	If known, membranous or muscular region may be defined (see 10187, 10193) 膜性または筋性の部位が分かるとき、明記される場合がある(10187、10193参照)	5-8
		Depression 陥没	*Diverticulum* 憩室	New	A non-patent localized recess in the membranous and muscular septum between the ventricles 心室中隔の膜性部あるいは筋性部における非開存性の局所的な陥凹		5-9
Aorta 大動脈	Aorta 大動脈	Overriding 騎乗		10205	Biventricular origin of aorta 大動脈が二心室にまたがり起始している		
	Aorta origin 大動脈起始部	Diverticulum 憩室	*Aneurism* 動脈瘤	New			

Table 1. List of Visceral Anomalies

Region / Organ / Structure	Observation		Synonym or *Related Term*	Ver. 1 Code No.	Definition	Note	Photo No.
Aorta 大動脈	Aorta origin 大動脈起始部	Malpositioned 位置異常		New	Outlet from heart displaced 心排出口の変位	See also Aorta, malpositioned 「大動脈、位置異常」項も参照	6-1
Aortic arch 大動脈弓	Aortic arch 大動脈弓	Absent 欠損		New			
		Atretic 閉鎖	Thread-like 索状	10206		May be total or partial 完全あるいは部分的な場合がある	
		Dilated 拡張(化)		10207		May be generalized or localized 全体あるいは局所の場合がある	
		Double 重複		New			
		High arched 高位		New	Aortic arch extends further upwards into neck 大動脈弓が頸部方向へかなり伸長している		
		Interrupted 離断		10208	Ascending aorta not connected to descending aorta 上行大動脈と下行大動脈がつながっていない		6-2
		Malpositioned 位置異常	*High-arched* *高位*	New		Use of related term 'high-arched' is recommended when arch extends further into neck 弓が頸部方向へかなり伸長している場合は、関連用語に記載された「高位（New）」を使用する	
		Narrow 狭窄		10209		May be generalized or localized 全体あるいは局所の場合がある	6-3
		Retroesophageal 食道背方		10210		Aortic arch usually passes behind trachea as well as esophagus この場合、大動脈弓は通常、食道と同様に気管の背側も走行する	6-4
		Right-sided 右側	Transposed 転換	10211			6-5

Table 1. List of Visceral Anomalies

Region / Organ / Structure	Observation		Synonym or *Related Term*	Ver. 1 Code No.	Definition	Note	Photo No.
Aortic arch 大動脈弓	Aortic arch 大動脈弓	Supernumerary branch 過剰起始	Supernumerary artery 動脈過剰	New	Additional artery arising from aortic arch 大動脈弓から起始している付加的な動脈		6-6
Artery 動脈	Artery 動脈	Supernumerary 過剰		New		General term for use if identity cannot be determined 識別できないときに使用する一般的な用語	6-7
Carotid artery 頸動脈	Carotid [May be further defined as common carotid, external, or internal] 頸動脈[総頸動脈、外頸動脈又は内頸動脈として定義される場合がある]	Absent 欠損		10212			
		Dilated 拡張(化)		10213		May be generalized or localized 全体あるいは局所の場合がある	
		Malpositioned 位置異常		10214	EC (Editor comment): With abnormal pass 編者注：走行に変化のあるもの	See also carotid artery origin, malpositioned. 「頸動脈起始部、位置異常」の項も参照	
		Narrow 狭窄		10215		May be generalized or localized. 全体あるいは局所の場合がある	
		Retroesophageal 食道背方		10216		Artery may pass behind trachea as well as esophagus 動脈は食道と同様に気管の背側も走行する場合がある	
		Supernumerary branch 過剰起始	Supernumerary artery 動脈過剰	New	Additional artery arising from carotid artery 頸動脈から起始している付加的な動脈		
Carotid artery 頸動脈	Carotid origin 頸動脈起始部	Malpositioned 位置異常		New	Origin (from aortic arch or innominate artery) of carotid artery, malpositioned. EC: Without abnormal pass 頸動脈の起始部(大動脈弓あるいは腕頭動脈からの発生部)、位置異常 編者注：走行に大きな変化のないもの	See also carotid artery, malpositioned 「頸動脈、位置異常」の項も参照 Includes carotid originating from aortic arch (i.e., absent innominate artery or common carotid trunk). 大動脈弓から起始する頸動脈もその一つである(例、腕頭動脈あるいは総頸動脈幹の欠損)	6-8

Table 1. List of Visceral Anomalies

Region / Organ / Structure	Observation		Synonym or Related Term	Ver. 1 Code No.	Definition	Note	Photo No.
Ductus arteriosus 動脈管	Ductus arteriosus 動脈管	Absent 欠損		10217			
		Atretic 閉鎖	Thread-like 索状	New		May be total or partial. 完全あるいは部分的な場合がある Normal after birth 生後は閉鎖するのが正常	
		Dilated 拡張(化)		10218		May be generalized or localized. 全体あるいは局所の場合がある	6-9
		Malpositioned 位置異常		10219	EC: With abnormal pass 編者注：走行に変化のあるもの	See also ductus arteriosus outlet, malpositioned. 「動脈管口、位置異常」の項も参照	
		Narrow 狭窄		10220		Normal occurrence after birth 生後は狭窄するのが正常	6-10
		Patent 開存	Persistent 遺残	10221	Open and unobstructed ductus arteriosus postnatally 生後も動脈管が開存している	Normal only in fetal period 胎児期のみ開存しているのが正常	
		Right-sided 右側	Transposed 転換	New			
Ductus arteriosus 動脈管	Ductus arteriosus outlet 動脈管口	Malpositioned 位置異常		New	Outlet (to aorta) from ductus arteriosus, malpositioned. 動脈管から動脈への流出口の位置異常	See also ductus arteriosus, malpositioned. 「動脈管、位置異常」の項も参照	
Great vessels 大血管	Great vessels 大血管	Fused vessel walls 血管壁癒合	Not separated 分離不全	New			
		Transposition 転換		10224	Origin of aorta from right ventricle and pulmonary trunk from left ventricle 大動脈は右心室から、肺動脈幹は左心室から起始している		6-11

Table 1. List of Visceral Anomalies

Region / Organ / Structure	Observation		Synonym or *Related Term*	Ver. 1 Code No.	Definition	Note	Photo No.
Great vessels 大血管	Aorticopulmonary septum 大動脈肺動脈中隔	Defect 欠損	Fistula; *confluence* 瘻；合流	10222	Communication between ascending aorta and pulmonary trunk 上行大動脈と肺動脈幹の間が通じている		
Great vessels 大血管	Truncus arteriosus 動脈幹	Persistent 遺残	Truncus arteriosus communis 総動脈幹(症)	10223	A common aortic and pulmonary trunk 大動脈と肺動脈幹が一本の動脈になっている		**6-12**
Innominate artery 腕頭動脈	Innominate artery (also known as brachiocephalic trunk) 腕頭動脈(無名動脈としても知られている)	Absent 欠損		New			
		Dilated 拡張(化)		10225			
		Long 伸長		10226			**6-13**
		Malpositioned 位置異常		10227	EC (Editor comment): With abnormal pass 編者注：走行に変化のあるもの	See also innominate artery origin, malpositioned. 「腕頭動脈起始部、位置異常」の項も参照	
		Narrow 狭窄		10228			
		Short 短小		10229			
		Supernumerary branch 過剰起始	Supernumerary artery 動脈過剰	New	Additional artery arising from innominate artery 腕頭動脈から起始している付加的な動脈	May be more than one 一本以上の場合がある	**6-14**
Innominate artery 腕頭動脈	Innominate artery origin 腕頭動脈起始部	Malpositioned 位置異常		New	Origin (from aortic arch) of innominate artery, malpositioned. EC: With abnormal pass 腕頭動脈の起始部(大動脈弓からの)、位置異常 編者注：走行に大きな変化のないもの	See also innominate artery, malpositioned. 「腕頭動脈、位置異常」の項も参照	

Table 1. List of Visceral Anomalies

Region / Organ / Structure	Observation		Synonym or *Related Term*	Ver. 1 Code No.	Definition	Note	Photo No.
Common Carotid Trunk 総頚動脈幹	Common carotid trunk 総頚動脈幹	Absent 欠損		New	Common trunk that divides into the innominate and left common carotid arteries. 腕頭動脈と左総頚動脈に分かれた総動脈管	Common carotid trunk is often present in rabbits, but there is no similar structure in normal rats 総頚動脈幹はウサギでよく見られるが、ラットでは同様の構造は見られない	
		Dilated 拡張(化)		New			
		Long 伸長		New			
		Malpositioned 位置異常		New	EC (Editor comment): With abnormal pass 編者注：走行に変化のあるもの	See also common carotid trunk origin, malpositioned. 「総頚動脈幹、位置異常」の項も参照	
		Narrow 狭窄		New			
		Present 有り		New		Abnormality in rats and mice ラットやマウスでは異常	
		Short 短小		New			
		Supernumerary branch 過剰起始	Supernumerary artery 動脈過剰	New	Additional artery arising from common carotid trunk 総頚動脈幹から起始している付加的な動脈		
Common Carotid Trunk 総頚動脈幹	Common carotid trunk origin 総頚動脈幹起始部	Malpositioned 位置異常		New	Origin (from aortic arch) of common carotid trunk, malpositioned. EC: Without abnormal pass 総頚動脈幹の起始部(大動脈弓からの)、位置異常、編者注：走行に大きな変化のないもの	See also common carotid trunk, malpositioned. 「総頚動脈幹、位置異常」の項も参照	
Pulmonary artery 肺動脈	Pulmonary artery 肺動脈	Absent 欠損		New			

Table 1. List of Visceral Anomalies

Region / Organ / Structure	Observation		Synonym or *Related Term*	Ver. 1 Code No.	Definition	Note	Photo No.
Pulmonary artery 肺動脈	Pulmonary artery 肺動脈	Atretic 閉鎖		New			
		Common origin 共通起始		New	Common origin of two arteries from pulmonary trunk 2本の肺動脈が肺動脈幹の同一部位から起始している		
		Dilated 拡張(化)		New			
		Malpositioned branch 起始異常		10230			
		Narrow 狭窄		New			
Pulmonary artery 肺動脈	Pulmonary artery origin 肺動脈起始部	Malpositioned 位置異常		New	Origin (from pulmonary trunk) of left/right pulmonary artery, malpositioned. EC (Editor comment): Without abnormal pass 左右肺動脈の起始部(肺動脈幹からの)、位置異常、編者注：走行に大きな変化のないもの		
Pulmonary trunk 肺動脈幹	Pulmonary trunk 肺動脈幹	Absent 欠損		New			
		Atretic 閉鎖	Thread-like 索状	10233		May be total or partial. 完全あるいは部分的な場合がある	
		Dilated 拡張(化)		10231			6-15
		Malpositioned 位置異常		New	EC: With abnormal pass 編者注：走行に変化のあるもの	See also pulmonary trunk origin, malpositioned. 「肺動脈幹起始部、位置異常」の項も参照	
		Narrow 狭窄		10232			6-16

Table 1. List of Visceral Anomalies

Region / Organ / Structure	Observation		Synonym or *Related Term*	Ver. 1 Code No.	Definition	Note	Photo No.
Pulmonary trunk 肺動脈幹	Pulmonary trunk 肺動脈幹	Retroesophageal 食道背方		10234		Pulmonary trunk may pass behind trachea as well as esophagus 肺動脈幹は食道と同様に気管の背側も走行する場合がある	
		Right-sided 右側		10235			
		Short 短小		New			
Pulmonary trunk 肺動脈幹	Pulmonary trunk origin 肺動脈幹起始部	Diverticulum 憩室	*Aneurism* *動脈瘤*	New			
		Malpositioned 位置異常		New	Outlet from heart displaced. 心臓からの起始異常	See also pulmonary trunk, malpositioned. 「肺動脈幹、位置異常」の項も参照	
Subclavian artery 鎖骨下動脈	Subclavian artery 鎖骨下動脈	Absent 欠損		10236			
		Dilated 拡張(化)		10237			
		Malpositioned 位置異常		10238	EC (Editor comment): With abnormal pass 編者注：走行に変化のあるもの	See also subclavian artery origin, malpositioned. 「鎖骨下動脈起始部、位置異常」の項も参照	6-17
		Narrow 狭窄		10239			
		Retroesophageal 食道背方		10240		Subclavian artery may pass behind trachea as well as esophagus 鎖骨下動脈は食道と同様に気管の背側も走行する場合がある	6-18
		Supernumerary 過剰		New			6-19

Table 1. List of Visceral Anomalies

Region / Organ / Structure	Observation		Synonym or *Related Term*	Ver. 1 Code No.	Definition	Note	Photo No.
Subclavian artery 鎖骨下動脈	Subclavian artery origin 鎖骨下動脈起始部	Malpositioned 位置異常		New	Origin (from aortic arch or innominate artery) of subclavian artery, malpositioned. EC (Editor comment): Without abnormal pass 鎖骨下動脈の起始部(大動脈弓あるいは腕頭動脈からの)、位置異常、編者注：走行に大きな変化のないもの	See also subclavian artery, malpositioned. 「鎖骨下動脈、位置異常」の項も参照 Includes right subclavian artery originating from aortic arch (i.e., absent innominate artery). 大動脈弓から起始する右鎖骨下動脈も含む(腕頭動脈欠損)	6-20
Umbilical artery 臍動脈	Umbilical artery 臍動脈	Absent 欠損		New		Note species differences. 種差に注意	
		Bilateral 両側		New		Normal in rabbits; Note species differences. ウサギでは正常；種差に注意	6-21
		Malpositioned 位置異常		New			
		Transposed 転換	*Left-sided* 左側	New		Note species differences. 種差に注意	6-22
Trachea 気管	Trachea 気管	Absent 欠損		New			
		Atretic 閉鎖		New		May be total or partial 完全あるいは部分的な場合がある	
		Collapsed lumen 虚脱管腔	Flat 扁平	New		May be generalized or localized 全体あるいは局所の場合がある	
		Dilated 拡張(化)		New		May be generalized or localized 全体あるいは局所の場合がある	
		Diverticulum 憩室		New			
		Fluid or other abnormal material 液体またはその他の異常物		New		May be an artifact アーティファクトの場合がある	
		Malpositioned 位置異常		10241			

Table 1. List of Visceral Anomalies

Region / Organ / Structure	Observation		Synonym or Related Term	Ver. 1 Code No.	Definition	Note	Photo No.
Trachea 気管	Trachea 気管	Narrow 狭窄		10242		May be generalized or localized 全体あるいは局所の場合がある	
Trachea 気管	Tracheoesophageal fistula 気管食道瘻			10243	Communication between esophageal and tracheal lumen 食道と気管の間の連絡		
Esophagus 食道	Esophagus 食道	Absent 欠損		10244			
		Atretic 閉鎖		10245		May be total or partial. 完全あるいは部分的な場合がある	
		Dilated 拡張(化)		New		May be generalized or localized. 全体あるいは局所の場合がある	
		Diverticulum 憩室		10246			
		Malpositioned 位置異常		10247			
		Narrow 狭窄		10248		May be generalized or localized. 全体あるいは局所の場合がある	
Lung 肺	Lung 肺	Abnormal lobation 分葉異常		10249	Global term for any abnormality （異常に対する）包括的な表現	Note species differences. 種差に注意 Further details of lobe(s) affected and change(s) observed may be specified in text. 影響のある葉を詳細に示す場合がある It is recommended that this global term is not used if individual lobes are routinely described in the laboratory. 個々の葉に言及する場合には本用語は使用しない	4-4
		Absent 欠損	Apulmonism 無肺(症)	10250			
		Large 大型(化)		10253			4-5
		Malpositioned 位置異常		10256			
		Misshapen 形態異常		10257			4-6
		Small 小型(化)		10259			4-7

Table 1. List of Visceral Anomalies

Region / Organ / Structure	Observation		Synonym or *Related Term*	Ver. 1 Code No.	Definition	Note	Photo No.
Lung 肺	Lobe [Affected lobe(s) should be specified; see also lung, abnormal lobation.] 葉 [影響のある葉を特定する； 「肺、分葉異常」の項も参照]	Absent 欠損		New			4-8
		Absent fissure 裂無形成		New			
		Cyst 嚢胞		New	Fluid-filled sac 液体が貯留した嚢		
		Fused 癒合	Not separated 分離不全	New			4-9
		Large 大型(化)		New			
		Malpositioned 位置異常		New			
		Misshapen 形態異常		New			
		Small 小型(化)		New			
		Supernumerary 過剰		10260		Note species differences. 種差に注意	4-10
		Supernumerary fissure 裂数過剰		New			
Veins 静脈	Anterior (cranial) vena cava 前(頭側)大静脈	Absent 欠損		10261			
		Dilated 拡張(化)		10264		May be generalized or localized 全体あるいは局所の場合がある	
		Interrupted 離断		10266			
		Malpositioned 位置異常		10268			
		Narrow 狭窄		10270		May be generalized or localized. 全体あるいは局所の場合がある	
Veins 静脈	Azygos vein 奇静脈	Absent 欠損		10262		Note species differences. 種差に注意	
		Bilateral 両側	Supernumerary, Persistent 過剰、遺残	10272	Azygos veins on both sides 両側奇静脈	Note species differences. 種差に注意	6-23

Table 1. List of Visceral Anomalies

Region / Organ / Structure	Observation		Synonym or Related Term	Ver. 1 Code No.	Definition	Note	Photo No.
Veins 静脈	Azygos vein 奇静脈	Malpositioned 位置異常		New		Not to be used as alternative to 10273 Transposed azygos vein 「10273 奇静脈転換」を除く	
		Persisting into abdomen 腹部遺残		New			
		Transposed 転換	Right-sided; Left-sided 右側；左側	10273	Azygos vein on opposite side from normal for species 正常の反対側にある奇静脈(動物種による)	Note species differences. 種差に注意	**6-24**
Veins 静脈	Posterior (caudal) vena cava 後(尾側)大静脈	Absent 欠損		10263			
		Branching variation 分岐変異		New	Variation in the branching of veins arising from the posterior vena cava 後大静脈から起始している静脈分岐の変異	May be further specified by location (position/laterality of branches) 位置を明確にした方がよい(分岐の位置/側性)	
		Dilated 拡張(化)		10265		May be generalized or localized 全体あるいは局所の場合がある	
		Interrupted 離断		10267			
		Malpositioned 位置異常		10269			**6-25**
		Narrow 狭窄		10271		May be generalized or localized 全体あるいは局所の場合がある	
Veins 静脈	Renal vein 腎静脈	Branched 分岐		New			
		Supernumerary 過剰	Doubled 重複	New			
Veins 静脈	Umbilical vein 臍静脈	Confluence with vena cava malpositioned 大静脈との位置異常		New			
		Malpositioned 位置異常		New			

Table 1. List of Visceral Anomalies

Region / Organ / Structure	Observation		Synonym or *Related Term*	Ver. 1 Code No.	Definition	Note	Photo No.
Veins 静脈	Vein 静脈	Supernumerary 過剰		New		May be used when the origin of supernumerary vein is uncertain 過剰を示した静脈の起始部が特定できない場合に使用する	
Diaphragm 横隔膜	Diaphragm 横隔膜	Absent 欠損		10274			
		Eventration 脱出	Protrusion of diaphragm 横隔膜の突出	10276	Abnormal anterior protrusion of a part of the diaphragm which is thin and covers variably displaced abdominal viscera 変位した腹部器官を覆っている横隔膜の一部が、薄くなって前方（胸腔）に突出している	May be generalized or localized 全体あるいは局所の場合がある	
		Hernia ヘルニア	Diaphragmatic hernia 横隔膜ヘルニア	10275	Absence of portion of the diaphragm with protrusion of some abdominal viscera into the thorax 腹腔内器官の胸腔への突出を伴う横隔膜の部分的欠損	Location (e.g., retrosternal, left/right posteriolateral) may be specified 位置（例、胸骨後、左/右の外後側部）を特定する場合がある	4-11
		Thin 菲薄		New	Generalized or localized thinning of diaphragm 全体あるいは局所に見られた菲薄化	If localized, region (muscular or tendinous) should be stated. Can be associated with raised area on surface of median liver lobe 局所であれば、部位（筋、腱）を特定する 肝臓表面の隆起に関連する	

Table 1. List of Visceral Anomalies

Region / Organ / Structure	Observation		Synonym or *Related Term*	Ver. 1 Code No.	Definition	Note	Photo No.
Liver 肝臓	Liver 肝臓	Abnormal lobation 分葉異常		New		Note species differences.　種差に注意 Further details of lobe(s) affected and change(s) observed may be specified in text. 影響のある葉を詳細に示す場合がある It is recommended that this global term is not used if individual lobes are routinely described in the laboratory. 個々の葉に言及する場合には本用語は使用しない	
		Absent 欠損		10278	Absence of entire organ 全器官の欠損		
		Discolored 変色	*Hepatorrhagia, Infarct* *肝出血, 梗塞(症)*	10279		May be generalized or localized 全体あるいは局所の場合がある "Infarct" to be used only if confirmed histologically 「梗塞」は病理組織学的に確認されたときのみ使用する	
		Large 大型(化)	Hepatomegaly 肝腫大	10281			
		Malpositioned 位置異常		10283			
		Misshapen 形態異常		10284			7-1
		Small 小型(化)	Microhepatia 小肝(症)	10286			
Liver 肝臓	Lobe [Affected lobe(s) should be specified; see also liver, abnormal lobation] 葉 [影響のある葉を特定する；「肝臓、分葉異常」の項も参照]	Absent 欠損		New	Absence of one or more lobes 1つ以上の肝分葉の欠損		7-2
		Additional fissure 過剰形成裂		New			7-3
		Cyst 嚢胞		New	Fluid-filled sac 液体が貯留した嚢		
		Fused 癒合	Not separated 分離不全	10277			
		Large 大型(化)		New			

Table 1. List of Visceral Anomalies

Region / Organ / Structure	Observation		Synonym or *Related Term*	Ver. 1 Code No.	Definition	Note	Photo No.
Liver 肝臓	Lobe 葉	Malpositioned 位置異常		New			
		Misshapen 形態異常		New			
		Small 小型(化)		New			
		Supernumerary 過剰		10287			**7-4**
Gallbladder / Bile Duct 胆嚢/胆管	Bile duct 胆管	Absent 欠損		10288			
		Long 伸長		10291			
		Malpositioned 位置異常		New		See also "Bile duct origin – Malpositioned" 「胆管起始部、位置異常」項も参照	
		Short 短小		10295			
		Supernumerary 過剰		New			
Gallbladder / Bile Duct 胆嚢/胆管	Bile duct origin 胆管起始部	Malpositioned 位置異常		New		See also "Bile duct - Malpositioned" 「胆管、位置異常」項も参照	
Gallbladder / Bile Duct 胆嚢/胆管	Gallbladder 胆嚢	Absent 欠損		10289		Note species differences. 種差に注意	
		Bilobed 二葉	*Bifurcated, Multilobed* 二分岐、多葉性	10290			**7-5**
		Diverticulum 憩室		New	Abnormal evagination 異常な膨出		
		Large 大型(化)		10292		Note species differences. 種差に注意	
		Malpositioned 位置異常		10293		Note species differences. 種差に注意	
		Misshapen 形態異常		10294		Note species differences. 種差に注意	
		Small 小型(化)		10296		Note species differences. 種差に注意	

Table 1. List of Visceral Anomalies

Region / Organ / Structure	Observation		Synonym or *Related Term*	Ver. 1 Code No.	Definition	Note	Photo No.
Gallbladder / Bile Duct 胆嚢/胆管	Gallbladder 胆嚢	Supernumerary 過剰		10297		Note species differences. 種差に注意	
Stomach 胃	Stomach 胃	Absent 欠損	Agastria 無胃症	10298			
		Atretic 閉鎖	Atretogastria 胃閉鎖症	10299		May be total or partial 完全あるいは部分的な場合がある	
		Cyst 嚢胞		New	Fluid-filled sac 液体が貯留した嚢		
		Distended 拡張(化)		10300	The structure of the stomach appears normal but it is distended due to abnormal contents 胃の形状は正常だが，異常な内容物により拡張している	Contents should be specified (e.g., gas, fluid) 内容物を特定する(例，ガス，液)	
		Diverticulum 憩室		10301			
		Large 大型(化)	Gastromegaly 胃巨大(症)	10302			
		Malpositioned 位置異常	Gastroptosis, Dextrogastria 胃下垂，右胃(症)	10303			
		Misshapen 形態異常		New			
		Narrow 狭窄		10304		Includes pylorus. 幽門を含む May be generalized or localized. 全体あるいは局所の場合がある	
		Small 小型(化)	Microgastria 小胃(症)	10305			
Pancreas 膵臓	Pancreas 膵臓	Absent 欠損		10306			
		Large 大型(化)		New			
		Malpositioned 位置異常		New			
		Small 小型(化)		10307			

Table 1. List of Visceral Anomalies

Region / Organ / Structure	Observation		Synonym or *Related Term*	Ver. 1 Code No.	Definition	Note	Photo No.
Pancreas 膵臓	Pancreas 膵臓	Supernumerary 過剰		10308			
Spleen 脾臓	Spleen 脾臓	Absent 欠損	Asplenia 無脾(症)	10309			
		Cyst 嚢胞		10310			
		Discolored 変色		10311		May be generalized or localized. 全体あるいは局所の場合がある	
		Large 大型(化)	Splenomegaly 脾臓腫大	10316			
		Malpositioned 位置異常		10312			
		Misshapen 形態異常		10313			
		Small 小型(化)	Microsplenia, *Narrow, Short* 小脾(症)，狭い，短い	10315			
		Split 分離	*Bipartite, Fragmented* 二分岐，断片(化)	New		May be divided into several small pieces 複数の小片に分離している場合がある	
		Supernumerary 過剰	Splenulus 副脾	10317			7-6
Intestines 腸	Intestine 腸	Absent 欠損		10318			7-7
		Atretic 閉鎖		10319		May be total or partial. 完全あるいは部分的な場合がある	
		Cyst 嚢胞		New			
		Distended 拡張(化)		New		Contents should be specified (e.g., gas, fluid) 内容物を特定する(例，ガス，液)	
		Diverticulum 憩室		10320			
		Fistula 瘻(孔)		10322			
		Interrupted 離断		New			

Table 1. List of Visceral Anomalies

Region / Organ / Structure		Observation	Synonym or Related Term	Ver. 1 Code No.	Definition	Note	Photo No.
Intestines 腸	Intestine 腸	Large 大型(化)	Enteromegaly 巨腸(症)	10321		May be generalized or localized. 全体あるいは局所の場合がある Content (e.g., gas, fluid) should be described, where appropriate. 内容物(例，ガス，液)を特定する	
		Malpositioned 位置異常		10323		May be generalized or localized. 全体あるいは局所の場合がある	7-8
		Narrow 狭窄		10324		May be generalized or localized. 全体あるいは局所の場合がある	
		Short 短小		10325			
Kidney 腎臓	Kidney 腎臓	Absent 欠損		10326			7-9
		Cyst 嚢胞		10328			7-10
		Discolored 変色	*Infarct* *梗塞(症)*	10330		May be generalized or localized 全体あるいは局所の場合がある 'Infarct' to be used only if confirmed histologically. 「梗塞」は病理組織学的に確認されたときのみ使用する Location within kidney (e.g., papilla, or cortex/medulla) may be specified 腎臓内の位置（例、乳頭、皮質/髄質）を特定する See also "Renal papilla – Discolored" 「腎乳頭、変色」項も参照	
		Large 大型(化)		10331			7-11
		Fused 癒合		10332			7-12
		Malpositioned 位置異常		10336			
		Misshapen 形態異常		10337			7-13
		Small 小型(化)		10339			7-14

Table 1. List of Visceral Anomalies

Region / Organ / Structure	Observation		Synonym or Related Term	Ver. 1 Code No.	Definition	Note	Photo No.
Kidney 腎臓	Kidney 腎臓	Supernumerary 過剰		10342		In some cases the separation of the duplicated organ may be incomplete 重複した器官の識別が困難な場合がある	
Kidney 腎臓	Renal pelvis 腎盂	Dilated 拡張(化)	*Distended*, *Hydronephrosis (10334)*, Renal pelvic cavitation 拡張, 水腎(症) (10334), 腎盂の腔化	10329	Hydronephrosis: Marked dilatation of renal pelvis and calices secondary to obstruction of urine flow, usually combined with destruction of the renal parenchyma 水腎：尿管の閉塞による二次的な腎盂や腎杯の顕著な拡張。通常、腎実質の崩壊を伴う	Dilated renal pelvis can be used for any severity detected at gross exam; hydronephrosis should be used in the most extreme cases. Destruction must be confirmed histopathologically. Often associated with dilated ureter (10358). 腎盂拡張は肉眼的に検査できる；水腎は極端な場合に使用する 腎実質の崩壊は病理組織学的に検査する しばしば、尿管拡張(10358)を伴う	7-15
		Small 小型(化)		10341			
Adrenal Gland 副腎	Adrenal 副腎	Absent 欠損		10343			7-16
		Discolored 変色		New		May be generalized or localized 全体あるいは局所の場合がある	7-17
		Fused 癒合		10346		Fused to another tissue 別組織との癒合	
		Large 大型(化)		10344			7-18
		Malpositioned 位置異常		10348			
		Misshapen 形態異常		10349			
		Small 小型(化)		10350			
		Supernumerary 過剰		10351			
Urinary Bladder 膀胱	Bladder 膀胱	Abnormal evagination 異常外転(反)	Diverticulum 憩室	New			

Table 1. List of Visceral Anomalies

Region / Organ / Structure	Observation		Synonym or *Related Term*	Ver. 1 Code No.	Definition	Note	Photo No.
Urinary Bladder 膀胱	Bladder 膀胱	Absent 欠損	Acystia 無膀胱(症)	10352			7-19
		Bilobed 二分葉	*Bifurcated* 分岐	New			
		Cyst 囊胞		10353			
		Distended 拡張(化)		10354		Contents should be specified (e.g., gas, fluid) 内容物を特定する(例，ガス，液)	7-20
		Misshapen 形態異常		New			
		Small 小型(化)		10355			
Ureter 尿管	Ureter 尿管	Absent 欠損		10356			7-21
		Atretic 閉鎖		New		May be total or partial 完全あるいは部分的な場合がある	
		Convoluted 蛇行	Coiled, Folded, Kinked, Twisted コイル状、褶曲、折れ、ねじれ	10357	Folded, curved, and/or tortuous windings 褶曲した、曲がった、ないしはねじれた尿管		7-22
		Dilated 拡張(化)	Hydroureter (10360) 尿管水腫(10360)	10358	Hydroureter: Abnormal distension of ureter with fluid, due to obstruction. 尿管水腫：閉鎖により尿管が液体で異常に膨張している	Dilated ureter can be used for any severity detected at gross exam; should note whether ureter is patent; hydroureter (see 10360) may be used in the most extreme cases and should be confirmed histopathologically Often associated with Dilated renal pelvis (10329) 尿管拡張は肉眼的に確認できる；尿管が閉鎖しているか確認する；尿管水腫(10360)は極端な場合に使用し、病理組織学的に確認する 通常、腎盂拡張(10329)を伴う	7-23
		Fused 癒合		New		May be total or partial 完全あるいは部分的な場合がある	

Table 1. List of Visceral Anomalies

Region / Organ / Structure	Observation		Synonym or *Related Term*	Ver. 1 Code No.	Definition	Note	Photo No.
Ureter 尿管	Ureter 尿管	Interrupted 離断		New			
		Malpositioned 位置異常		New		Excludes Retrocaval ureter. See also 10361 大静脈背方尿管を除く 10361も参照	
		Narrow 狭窄		New		May be generalized or localized 全体あるいは局所の場合がある	
		Supernumerary 過剰		10359			
		Retrocaval 大静脈背方		10361	Passing dorsally to the vena cava 尿管が大静脈の背方を走行している	See also above Malpositioned ureter 「尿管、位置異常」も参照	
		Short 短小		New			
Gonad 生殖腺	Gonads 生殖腺	Absent 欠損		10362		Used when sex cannot be determined 性が判定できない場合に用いる	
	Hermaphroditism (真性)半陰陽		Hermaphrodism (真性)半陰陽	10363	Presence of both male and female gonadal tissue 雌雄の両生殖腺組織を有する		
	Pseudoherma- phroditism 仮性半陰陽		Pseudoherma- phrodism 仮性半陰陽	New	Gonads of one sex are present, while the external genital organs resemble in the opposite sex 雌雄いづれかの生殖腺を持つが，外生殖器は異なる性を示す		
Testis 精巣	Testis 精巣	Absent 欠損	Anorchia 無睾丸(症)	10366		If both gonads are absent and sex cannot be determined, use "Absent gonads" – see 10362 両側欠損で性別が判定できない場合は「生殖腺欠損」(10362参照)を用いる	8-1
		Cyst 嚢胞		New			
		Large 大型(化)		10367			

Table 1. List of Visceral Anomalies

Region / Organ / Structure	Observation		Synonym or Related Term	Ver. 1 Code No.	Definition	Note	Photo No.
Testis 精巣	Testis 精巣	Malpositioned 位置異常		10369	Testis not descended to lower pelvic region or (postnatally) into the scrotum 精巣が骨盤あるいは陰嚢内まで下降していない		8-2
		Misshapen 形態異常		10370			
		Small 小型(化)		10371			
		Supernumerary 過剰		10372			
Ovary 卵巣	Ovary 卵巣	Absent 欠損		10382		If both gonads are absent use "Absent gonads" – see 10362 両側欠損の場合は「生殖腺欠損」(10362参照)を用いる	
		Cyst 嚢胞		10383			
		Discolored 変色	*Oophorrhagia* 排卵性出血	New		Specify color 色を特定する	
		Large 大型(化)		10384			
		Malpositioned 位置異常		10386			8-3
		Misshapen 形態異常		10387			
		Small 小型(化)		10388			
		Supernumerary 過剰		10389			
Uterus 子宮	Uterus 子宮	Atretic 閉鎖	Hysteratresia 子宮閉鎖（症）	10398		May be total or partial 完全あるいは部分的な場合がある	
		Cyst 嚢胞		New			
		Dilated 拡張(化)	Distended 拡張	New			

Table 1. List of Visceral Anomalies

Region / Organ / Structure	Observation		Synonym or *Related Term*	Ver. 1 Code No.	Definition	Note	Photo No.
Uterus 子宮	Uterus 子宮	Interrupted 離断		New			
		Large 大型(化)		New	One or both horns increased in size 片側または両側の子宮角の大型化	May be generalized or localized 全体あるいは局所の場合がある	
		Long 伸長		New	One or both horns increased in length 片側または両側の子宮角の伸張		
		Misshapen 形態異常		10400			
		Narrow 狭窄		New		May be generalized or localized 全体あるいは局所の場合がある	**8-4**
		Small 小型(化)		10401	One or both horns reduced in size 片側または両側の子宮角の小型化	May be generalized or localized 全体あるいは局所の場合がある	**8-5**
Uterus 子宮	Uterus horn 子宮角	Absent 欠損		10397		May be unilateral or bilateral 片側性あるいは両側性がある	**8-6**

Table 2 Comparative List of This Atlas Findings, Mouse Phenotype, and Human Phenotype

Photo No.	Atlas Term	MP No.	MP Term	HP No.	HP Term
1-1	Situs inversus (total) 内臓逆位(胸腹部)	0011252	Situs inversus totalis	0001696	Situs inversus totalis
2-1	Misshapen brain (Dupuricated brain) 脳形態異常(重複脳)	0002152	Abnormal brain morphology	0012443	Abnormality of brain morphology
2-2	Misshapen cerebrum 大脳形態異常	0008540	Abnormal cerebrum morphology	0002060	Abnormality of the cerebrum
2-3	Dilated lateral (cerebral) ventricule 側脳室拡張	0000825	Dilated lateral ventricles	0006956	Dilation of lateral ventricles
2-4	Large perimeningeal space 髄膜周辺腔拡張(化)				
2-5	Dilated third ventricle of the brain 第三脳室拡張	0000827	Dilated third ventricle	0007082	Dilated third ventricle
3-1	Absent eye (Anophthalmia) 眼欠損(無眼球)	0001293	Anophthalmia	0000528	Anophthalmia
3-2	Small eye (Micropthalmia) 眼小型(小眼球)	0001297	Microphthalmia	0000568	Microphthalmos
3-3	Msshapen lens 水晶体形態異常	0001303	Abnormal lens morphology	0011526	Abnormality of lens shape
3-4	Opacity of the lens 水晶体混濁	0001304	Cataracts	0000519	Congenital cataract
3-5	Fold retina 網膜皺襞	0003727	Abnormal retinal layer morphology	0008052	Abnormal retinal folds
3-6	Large nasal cavity 鼻腔大型(化)	0002237	Abnormal nasal cavity morphology	0010640	Abnormality of the nasal cavity
3-7	Small nasal cavity 鼻腔小型(化)	0002237	Abnormal nasal cavity morphology	0010640	Abnormality of the nasal cavity
3-8	Absent nasal septum 鼻中隔欠損	0004872	Absent nasal septum	0009935	Aplasia/Hypoplasia of the nasal septum
4-1	Thymic cord 胸腺索	0010722	Persistent cervical thymus	0010517	Ectopic thymus tissue
4-2	Misshapen thymus 胸腺形態異常	0000703	Abnormal thymus morphology	0000777	Abnormality of the thymus
4-3	Small thymus 胸腺小型(化)	0000706	Small thymus	0000778	Hypoplasia of the thymus
4-4	Abnormal lobation of the lung 肺分葉異常	0010975	Abnormal lung lobe morphology	0002101	Abnormal lung lobation
4-5	Large lung 肺大型(化)	0004882	Enlarged lung		
4-6	Misshapen lung 肺形態異常	0001175	Abnormal lung morphology	0002088	Abnormality of the lung
4-7	Small lung 肺小型(化)	0003641	Small lung	0002089	Pulmonary hypoplasia
4-8	Absent lung lobe 肺葉欠損	0011011	Impaired lung lobe morphogenesis		
4-9	Fused lung lobe 肺葉癒合	0010977	Fused right lung lobes		
4-10	Supernumerary lobes of the lung 肺葉過剰	0010975	Abnormal lung lobe morphology	0002101	Abnormal lung lobation
4-11	Diaphragmatic hernia 横隔膜ヘルニア	0003924	Herniated diaphragm	0000776	Congenital diaphragmatic hernia
5-1	Atrial septum defect 心房中隔欠損	0010403	Atrial septum defect	0001631	Defect in the atrial septum
5-2	Persistent atrioventricular (A-V) canal 共通房室口遺残	0010412	Atrioventricular septal defect	0001674	Complete atrioventricular canal defect
5-3	Premature closure of foramen ovale 卵円孔早期閉鎖				
5-4	Misshapen heart 心臓形態異常	0000277	Abnormal heart shape		
5-5	Misshapen left atrioventricular (A-V) valve 左房室弁形態異常	0000286	Abnormal mitral valve morphology	0001633	Abnormality of the mitral valve
5-6	Misshapen pulmonary valve 肺動脈弁形態異常	0002748	Abnormal pulmonary valve morphology	0001641	Abnormality of the pulmonary valve

MP: Mouse phenotype
HP: Human phenotype
In some cases, MP and HP terms indicate a more general description for the Atlas term.

Table 2 Comparative List of This Atlas Findings, Mouse Phenotype, and Human Phenotype

Photo No.	Atlas Term	MP No.	MP Term	HP No.	HP Term
5-7	Double outlet from the right ventricle 両大血管起始(右室)	0000284	Double outlet right ventricle (DORV)	0001719	Double outlet right ventricle
5-8	Ventricular septum defect 心室中隔欠損	0010402	Ventricular septal defect	0001629	Ventricular septal defect
5-9	Depression of ventricular septum 心室中隔陥没	0020136	Abnormal interventricular seputum thickness	0010438	Abnormality of the ventricular septum
6-1	Malpositioned aorta origin 大動脈起始部位置異常	0010426	Abnormal heart and great artery attachment	0011563	Abnormal ventriculo-arterial connection
6-2	Interrupted aortic arch 大動脈弓離断	0004157 0010469	Interrupted aortic arch Ascending aorta hypoplasia	0011611	Interrupted aortic arch
6-3	Narrow aortic arch 大動脈弓狭窄	0010526	Aortic arch coarctation	0005151	Preductal coarctation of the aorta
6-4	Retroesophageal aortic arch 食道背方大動脈弓	0010466	Vascular ring	0010775	Vascular ring
6-5	Right-sided aortic arch 右側大動脈弓	0004158	Right aortic arch	0012020	Right aortic arch
6-6	Supernumerary branch from the aortic arch 大動脈弓過剰起始	0004113	Abnormal aortic arch morphology	0011587	Abnormal branching pattern of the aortic arch
6-7	Supernumerary artery 動脈過剰	0010472	Abnormal ascending aorta and coronary artery attachment	0011636	Abnormal origin of the coronary arteries
6-8	Malpositioned carotid origin 頸動脈起始部位置異常	0010464	Abnormal aortic arch and aortic arch branch attachment	0011587	Abnormal branching pattern of the aortic arch
6-9	Dilated ductus arteriosus 動脈管拡張(化)	0010564	Abnormal fetal ductus arteriosus morphology		
6-10	Narrow ductus arteriosus 動脈管狭窄	0010564	Abnormal fetal ductus arteriosus morphology		
6-11	Transposition of great vesseles 大血管転換	0004110	Transposition of great artrries	0001669	Transposition of the great arteries
6-12	Persistent truncus arteriosus 動脈幹遺残	0002633	Persistent truncus arteriosus	0001660	Truncus arteriosus
6-13	Long innominate artery 腕頭動脈伸長				
6-14	Supernumerary branch from the innominate artery 腕頭動脈過剰起始				
6-15	Dilated pulmonary trunk 肺動脈幹拡張(化)	0010649	Dilated pulmonary trunk		
6-16	Narrow pulmonary trunk 肺動脈幹狭窄	0010459	Supravalvar pulmonary trunk stenosis		
6-17	Malpositioned subclavian artery 鎖骨下動脈位置異常				
6-18	Retroesophageal right subclavian artery 食道背方右鎖骨下動脈	0004160	Retroesophagea right subclavian artery	0011595	Left aortic arch with retroesophageal right subclavian artery
6-19	Supernumerary subclavian artery 鎖骨下動脈過剰	0004113	Abnormal aortic arch morphology	0011587	Abnormal branching pattern of the aortic arch

MP: Mouse phenotype
HP: Human phenotype
In some cases, MP and HP terms indicate a more general description for the Atlas term.

Table 2 Comparative List of This Atlas Findings, Mouse Phenotype, and Human Phenotype

Photo No.	Atlas Term	MP No.	MP Term	HP No.	HP Term
6-20	Malpositioned subclavian artery origin 鎖骨下動脈起始部位置異常	0010465	Aberrant origin of the right subclavian artery	0011587	Abnormal branching pattern of the aortic arch
6-21	Bilateral umbilical artery 両側臍動脈	0003230	Abnormal umbilical artery morphology		
6-22	Transposed umbilical artery 臍動脈転換	0003230	Abnormal umbilical artery morphology		
6-23	Bilateral azygos veins 両側奇静脈	0011569	Abnormal azygos vein morphology		
6-24	Transposed azygos vein 奇静脈転換	0011569	Abnormal azygos vein morphology		
6-25	Malpositioned posterior (caudal) vena cava 後(尾側)大静脈位置異常	0006063	Abnormal inferior vena cava morphology	0005345	Abnormality of the vena cava
7-1	Misshapen liver 肝臓形態異常	0000598	Abnormal liver morphology	0100752	Abnormal liver lobulation
7-2	Absent lobe of the liver 肝臓葉欠損	0000598	Abnormal liver morphology	0100752	Abnormal liver lobulation
7-3	Additional fissure of the liver 肝臓葉過剰形成裂				
7-4	Supernumerary lobes of the liver 肝臓葉過剰	0000598	Abnormal liver morphology	0100752	Abnormal liver lobulation
7-5	Bilobed gallbladder 胆嚢二葉	0005084	Abnormal gallbladder morphology	0005608	Bilobate gallbladder
7-6	Supernumerary spleen 脾臓過剰	0003342	Accessory spleen	0001747	Accessory spleen
7-7	Absent intestine 腸欠損				
7-8	Malpositioned intestine 腸位置異常	0005155 0006077	Herniated intestine Inguinal hernia	0004299 0000023	Hernia of the abdominal wall Inguinal hernia
7-9	Absent kidney 腎臓欠損	0000520	Absent kidney	0000104	Renal agenesis
7-10	Cyst in the kidney 腎臓嚢胞	0003675	Kidney cysts	0000107	Renal cyst
7-11	Large kidney 腎臓大型(化)	0003068	Enlarged kidney	0000105	Enlarged kidneys
7-12	Fused kidney 腎臓癒合	0003605	Fused kidneys	0004736 0000085	Crossed fused renal ectopia Horseshoe kidney
7-13	Misshapen kidney 腎臓形態異常	0002135	Abnormal kidney morphology	0012210	Abnormal renal morphology
7-14	Small kidney 腎臓小型(化)	0002989	Small kidney	0000089	Renal hypoplasia
7-15	Dilated renal pelvis 腎盂拡張	0000519	Hydronephrosis	0010946 0010945	Dilatation of the renal pelvis Fetal pyelectasis
7-16	Absent adrenal 副腎欠損	0005313	Absent adrenal gland	0011743	Adrenal gland agenesis
7-17	Discolored adrenal 副腎変色				
7-18	Large adrenal 副腎大型(化)	0000642 0009078	Enlarged adrenal glands Adrenal gland hyperplasia	0008258	Congenital adrenal hyperplasia
7-19	Absent urinary bladder 膀胱欠損	0009252	Absent urinary bladder	0010477	Aplasia of the bladder
7-20	Distended urinary bladder 膀胱拡張	0000539	Distended urunary bladder	0010955	Dilatation of the bladder
7-21	Absent ureter 尿管欠損	0003722	Absent ureter	0012300	Ureteral agenesis
7-22	Convoluted ureter 尿管蛇行	0000534	Abnormal ureter morphology	0000069	Abnormality of the ureter

MP: Mouse phenotype
HP: Human phenotype
In some cases, MP and HP terms indicate a more general description for the Atlas term.

Table 2 Comparative List of This Atlas Findings, Mouse Phenotype, and Human Phenotype

Photo No.	Atlas Term	MP No.	MP Term	HP No.	HP Term
7-23	Dilated ureter 尿管拡張	0003586 0000536	Dilated ureter Hydroureter	0000072	Hydroureter
8-1	Absent testes 精巣欠損	0006415	Absent testes	0010469	Aplasia of the testes
8-2	Malpositioned testis 精巣位置異常	0011410	Ectopic testis	0000028	Cryptorchidism
8-3	Malpositioned ovary 卵巣位置異常	0011727	Ectopic ovary		
8-4	Narrow uterus 子宮狭窄	0003572	Abnormal uterus development		
8-5	Small uterus 子宮小型化	0002637	Small uterus	0000013	Hypoplasia of the uterus
8-6	Absent uterine horn 子宮角欠損	0003558	Absent uterus	0000151	Aplasia of the uterus

MP: Mouse phenotype
HP: Human phenotype
In some cases, MP and HP terms indicate a more general description for the Atlas term.

Photographs of Normal Fetuses in Rats
正常写真（ラット）

Head

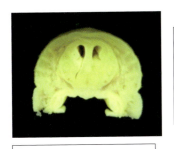

Section 1 of the head

Nasal cavities and septum can be observed.
鼻（鼻腔及び鼻中隔）が観察できる。

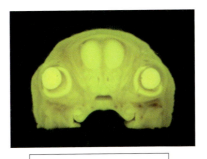

Section 2 of the head

Olfactory lobes and eyes can be observed.
嗅葉及び眼が観察できる。

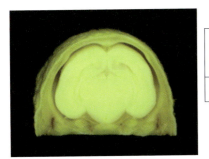

Section 3 of the head

Cerebrum and ventricles can be observed.
大脳及び脳室が観察できる。

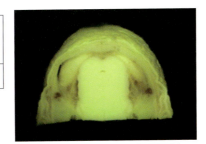

Section 4 of the head

Cerebellum and inner/middle ears can be observed.
小脳及び耳が観察できる。

Thoracic cavity

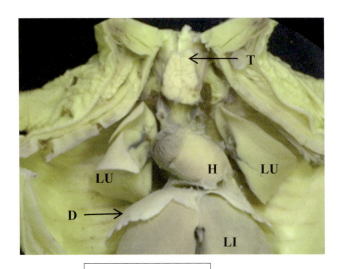

Thoracic cavity

Thymus, heart, lung and diaphragm can be observed.
胸腺、心臓、肺、横隔膜が観察できる。

T: Thymus   H: Heart
LU: Lung   D: Diaphragm
LI: Liver

Heart

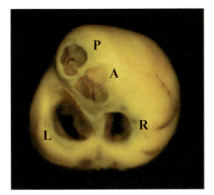

Outward view

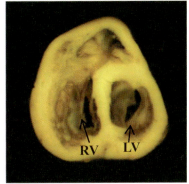

Internal view

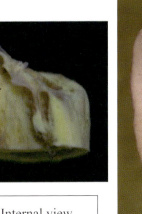

Internal view

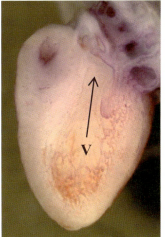

Position and size of aorta, pulmonary trunk, and right and left atrioventricular ostium, and shape of aortic valve, pulmonary valve, and right and left atrioventricular valves can be observed.

大動脈、肺動脈幹、左右房室口の位置、大きさ及び大動脈弁、肺動脈弁、左右房室弁が観察できる。

A: Aorta
P: Pulmonary trunk
R: Right atrioventricular ostium
L: Left atrioventricular ostium
RV: Right atrioventricular valve
LV: Left atrioventricular valve
V: Ventricular septum (Membranous)

Membranous ventricular septum can be observed.

心室中隔（膜性部）が観察できる。

Abdominal cavity

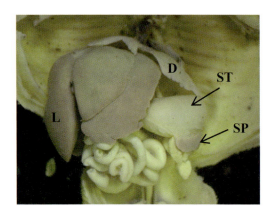

Diaphragm, liver, spleen, stomach, and intestine can be observed.

横隔膜、肝臓、脾臓、胃、腸管が観察できる。

D: Diaphragm
L: Liver
ST: Stomach
SP: Spleen
K: Kidney
UR: Ureter
O: Ovary
UT: Uterus
T: Testis

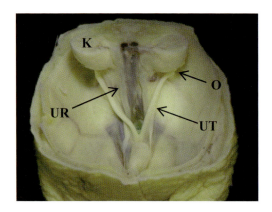

Female

Kidney, ureter, ovary (left photo), uterus (left photo) and testis (right photo) can be observed.

腎臓、尿管、卵巣（左図）、子宮（左図）及び精巣（右図）が観察できる。

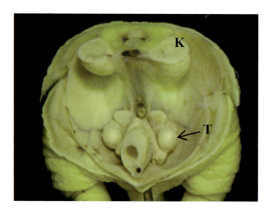

Male

Photographs of Visceral Anomalies

1. General

1-1　Situs inversus (total)　内臓逆位（胸腹部）　(10127)

Species	Rat
Memo	Situs inversus (total): Mirror-image transposition of the thoracic and abdominal viscera.
	内臓逆位（胸腹部）：胸部と腹部の器官の位置が正常に対して鏡像的に逆になっている。

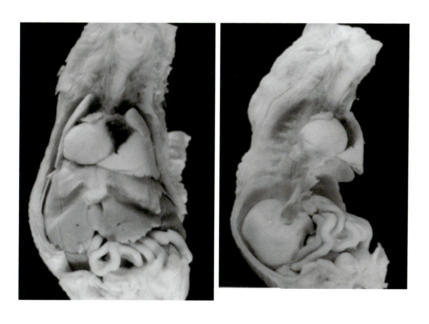
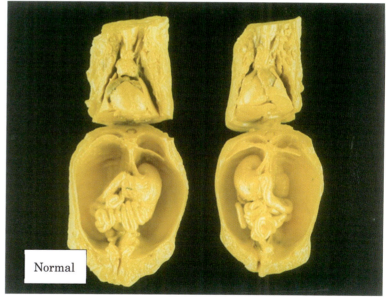

Photographs of Visceral Anomalies

2. Brain

2-1 Misshapen brain (Duplicated brain) 脳形態異常（重複脳）(New)

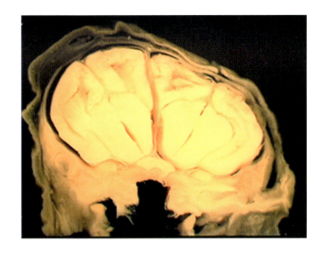

Species	Rat
Memo	Misshapen brain, Duplicated brain: This fetus is considered to be "Conjoined twins".
	脳形態異常、重複脳：脳が重複している。二重体の一種と考えられる。

2-2 Misshapen cerebrum　大脳形態異常　(10133)

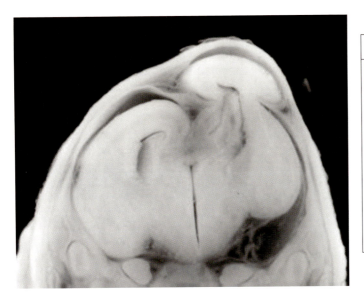

Species	Rat
Memo	Misshapen cerebrum: The brain, ventricle and meninges herniate through a cranial opening. This is "Meningohydro-encephalocele (New)" in external examination. This external finding can be confirmed by this section although it is difficult to distinguish "Meningohydro-encephalocele (New)" from "Meningoencephalocele (10017)" in external examination.
	大脳形態異常：頭蓋の開口により髄膜と脳室の一部を含む脳が突出している。外表の観察では髄膜水脳瘤（New）と髄膜脳瘤（10017）は区分し難いが、この断面により髄膜水脳瘤と判断できる。

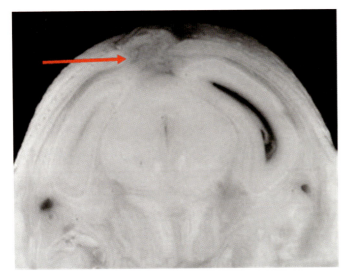

Species	Rat
Memo	Misshapen cerebrum: The meninges herniate through defect in skull. This is cranial meningocele (10016) in external examination.
	大脳形態異常：頭骨の一部が欠損し、髄膜が突出している。外表では頭蓋髄膜瘤（10016）

2-3 Dilated lateral (cerebral) ventricle　側脳室拡張　(10128)

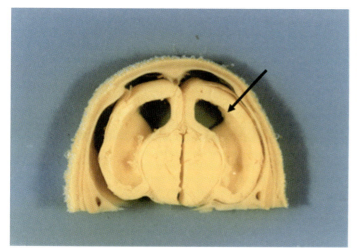

Species	Rat, SD
Memo	Dilated lateral (cerebral) ventricle: Internal hydrocephaly (10131 in Ver.1).
	側脳室拡張：内水頭症(Ver.1：10131)とも言う。

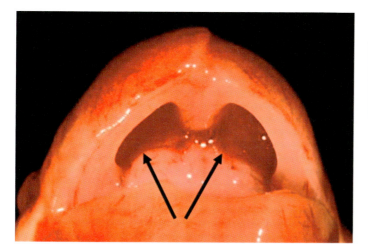

Species	Rabbit
Memo	Dilated lateral (cerebral) ventricle: Internal hydrocephaly (10131 in Ver.1)
	側脳室拡張：内水頭症（Ver.1：10131）とも言う。

2-3 Continued

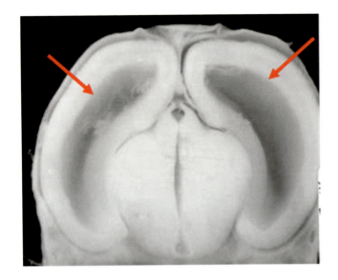

Species	Rat, SD
Memo	Dilated lateral (cerebral) ventricle: Internal hydrocephaly (10131 in Ver.1).
	側脳室拡張：内水頭症(Ver.1：10131)とも言う。

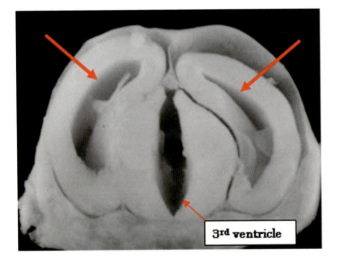

Species	Rat
Memo	Dilated lateral ventricle of the brain with Dilated third ventricle (New): Internal hydrocephaly (10131 in Ver.1)
	側脳室拡張：第三脳室も拡張（New）。内水頭症（Ver.1では10131）とも言う。

2-4 Large perimeningeal space 髄膜周辺腔拡張（化） (New)

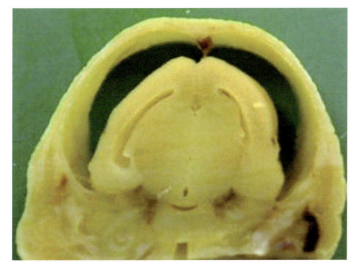

Species	Rat
Memo	Large perimeningeal space: This finding is "External hydrocephaly (10131) in Ver. 1.
	髄膜周辺腔拡張（化）：Ver. 1 では外水頭症（10131）

2-5 Dilated third ventricle of the brain　第三脳室拡張　(New)

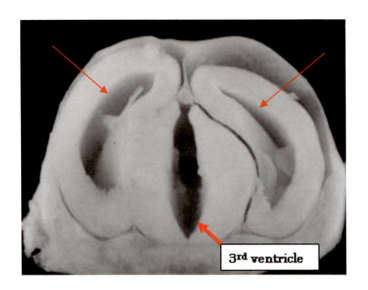

Species	Rat
Memo	Dilated third ventricle of the brain with Dilated lateral ventricle (10128): Internal hydrocephaly (10131 in Ver.1)
	第三脳室拡張：側脳室も拡張（10128）。内水頭症（Ver.1 では 10131）とも言う。

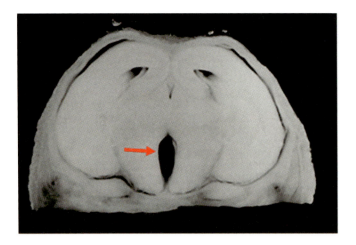

Species	Rat
Memo	Dilated third ventricle of the brain
	第三脳室拡張

Photographs of Visceral Anomalies

3. Eye and Nose

3-1 Absent eye (Anophthalmia) 眼欠損（無眼球） (10137)

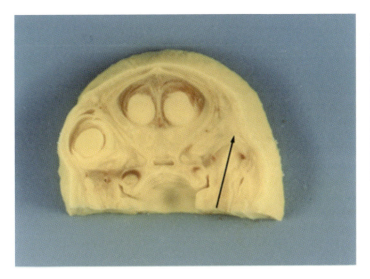

Species	Rat, SD
Memo	Absent eye or Anophthalmia: The eye tissues (structures) cannot be confirmed by observation with a stereomicroscope.
	眼欠損（無眼球）：肉眼観察において、眼の組織（構造）が認められない。可能であれば、病理組織学的確認が望まれるが、実務上肉眼での判断は許容される。

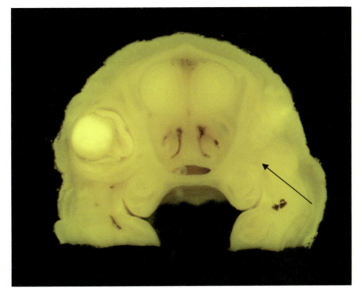

Species	Rat
Memo	Absent eye or Anophthalmia: The eye tissues (structures) cannot be confirmed by observation with a stereomicroscope.
	眼欠損（無眼球）：肉眼観察において、眼の組織が認められない。

3-2 Small eye   眼小型   (10143)

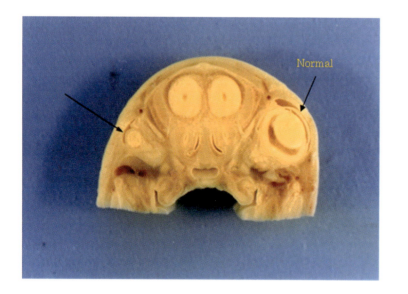

Species	Rat, SD
Memo	Small eye or Microphthalmia: The left eye is small.
	眼小型（化）、小眼球（症）：眼球全体が小さい。

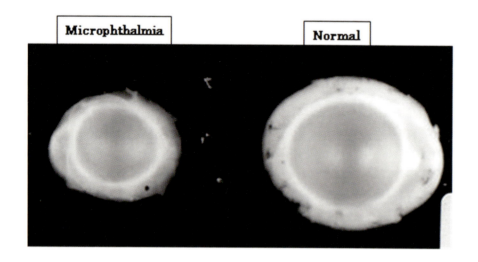

Species	Rabbit
Memo	Small eye or Microphthalmia: Smaller than the normal eye (Right fig.)
	眼小型（化）、小眼球（症）：正常（右図）に比べ眼球が小さい。

3-2 Continued

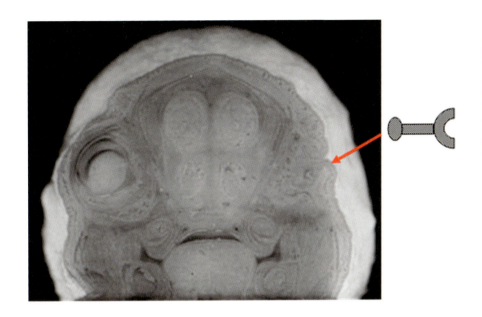

Species	Rat
Memo	Small eye or Microphthalmia: Underdeveloped eye tissues (structures) can be confirmed.
	眼小型（化）、小眼球（症）：未発生（退縮）の眼組織（眼杯構造）が確認できる。

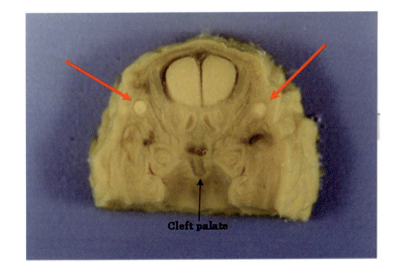

Species	Rat, SD
Memo	Small eye, Microphthalmia: Both eyeballs are small. This fetus has externally "Cleft palate (10052)".
	眼小型（化）、小眼球（症）：両眼が小さい。外表観察では口蓋裂（10052）を伴う。

3-3 Misshapen lens 水晶体形態異常 (10144)

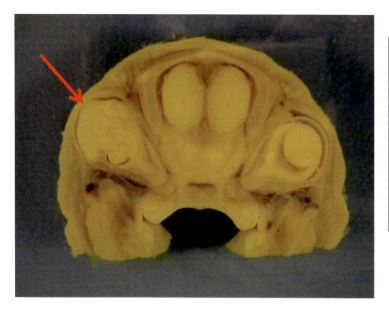

Species	Rat, SD
Memo	Misshapen lens: Structures of the whole eye including lens and retina are abnormal. Although "Misshapen eye" is better term, this name is used because the term "Misshapen eye" is not in the harmonized terminology of the developmental anomalies.
	水晶体形態異常：水晶体、網膜を含め、眼全体の形態が異常である。眼形態異常と言う所見が妥当であるが、統一用語には「眼形態異常」がないので、ここに掲載する。

3-4　Opacity of the lens　水晶体混濁　(10139)

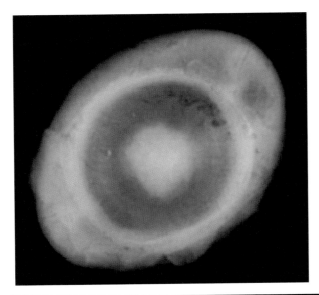

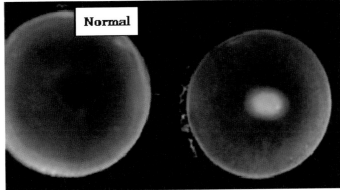

Species	Rabbit
Memo	Opacity of the lens or Cataract: Opacity of the crystalline lens is observed. This is an artifact when the opacity disappears after soaking in warm water (about 37℃). This artifactual opacity is due to diminished light transmission due to decreased temperature and cell contraction in the lens.
	水晶体混濁、白内障：水晶体が白く混濁している。アーティファクト（胎児体温低下による光透過性の低下）によることもあり、注意する必要がある。37℃程度の温水に浸け、消えればアーティファクト。

3-5　Fold retina　網膜皺襞　(10146)

Species	Rat, SD
Memo	Fold retina: Undulation of retinal layers (arrow)
	網膜皺襞：網膜の一部が波状になっている（矢印）。

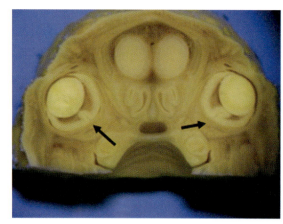
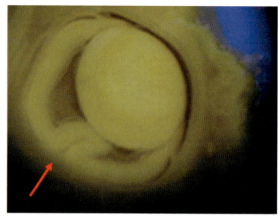

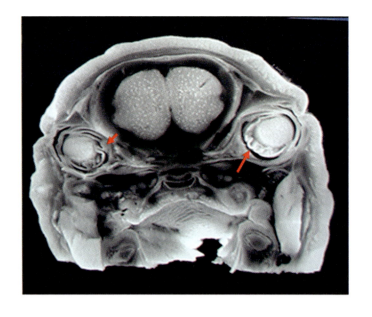

Species	Rabbit
Memo	Fold retina: Undulation of retinal layers (arrow).
	網膜皺襞：網膜の一部が波状になっている（矢印）。

3-6　Large nasal cavity　鼻腔大型（化）　(10150)

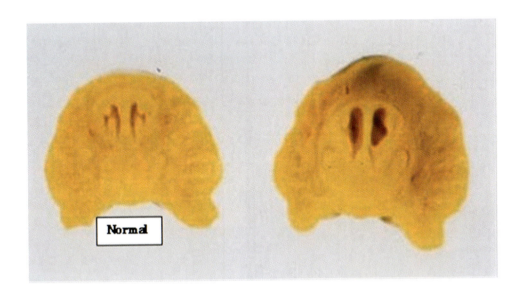

Species	Rat
Memo	Large nasal cavity
	鼻腔大型（化）

3-7　Small nasal cavity　鼻腔小型（化）　(10153)

Species	Rat
Memo	Small nasal cavity: The left nasal cavity is small. The top of the nose is slightly different in size. It may be possible that this is "Misshapen nasal cavity (New)".
	鼻腔小型（化）：左鼻腔が小さい。外表観察では鼻先端（球部）の大きさに若干の左右差がある。鼻腔形態異常（New）でも良い。

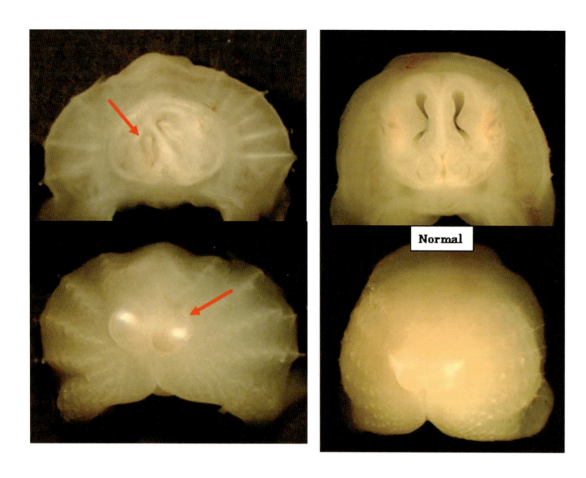

3-8 Absent nasal septum 鼻中隔欠損 (10149)

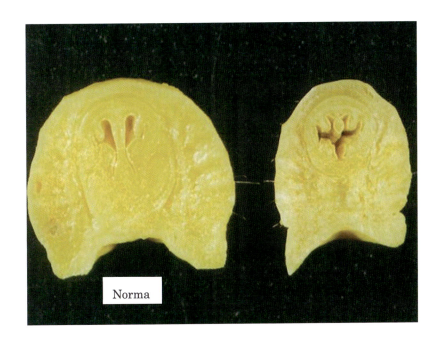

Species	Rat
Memo	Absent nasal septum
	鼻中隔欠損

Photographs of Visceral Anomalies

4. Thoracic Organs

4-1　Thymic cord　胸腺索　(New)

Species	Rat, SD
Memo	Thymic cord, Thymic remnant in the neck or Extra thymic tissue: The horn of the thymus is undescended partially (black arrow).
	胸腺索：胸腺頸部残留、あるいは、胸腺組織過剰とも言う。部分的な胸腺の下降不全で、一部が頭部方向に長い。

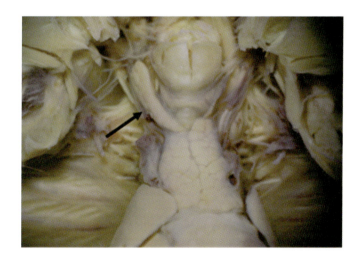 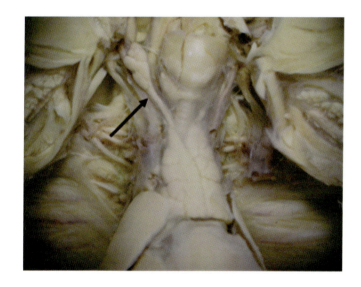

4-2 Misshappen thymus　胸腺形態異常　(10161)

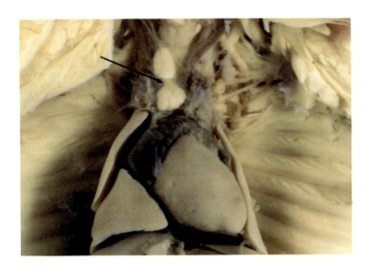

Species	Rat, SD
Memo	Misshappen thymus: Reduced size and indistinct lobe formation in the right and left sides of the thymus that also has narrow isthmus (black arrow) at the middle position.
	胸腺形態異常：全体として小さく、左右の葉が不明確。上下の中間にくびれが見られる。

4-3 Small thymus　胸腺小型（化）　(10162)

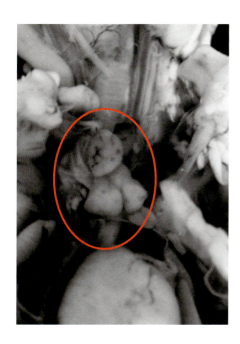

Species	Rabbit
Memo	Small thymus: The thymus is smaller than normal.
	胸腺小型

4-4 Abnormal lobation of the lung 肺分葉異常 (10249)

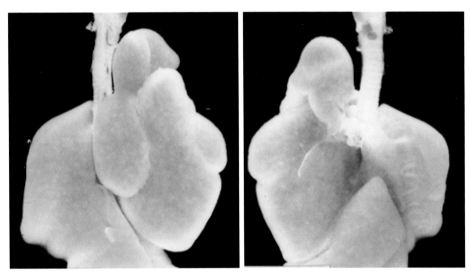

Dorsal view   Ventral view

Species	Rabbit
Memo	Abnormal lobation of the lung: Lung lobation is generally abnormal; Shape and number.
	肺分葉異常：全体的（形、数）に肺の分葉が異常。

4-5 Large lung 肺大型（化） (10253)

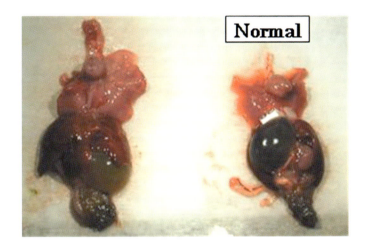

Species	Rabbit
Memo	Large lung: The lung is generally big compared with normal lung. The trachea may also be enlarged.
	肺大型（化）：全体的に正常に比べ大きい。気管も太い。

4-6 Misshapen lung 肺形態異常 (10257)

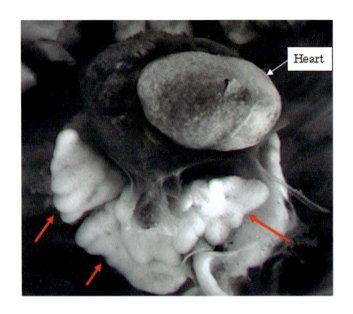

Species	Rabbit
Memo	Misshapen lung: The development of the lung is delayed and its shape is the same as the lung bud (arrow).
	肺形態異常：肺の発生が遅延し、肺芽様の形態がみられる（矢印）。

4-7 Small lung 肺小型（化） (10259)

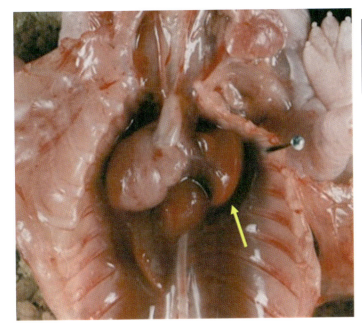

Species	Rabbit
Memo	Small lung: The lung is generally small, and the left lobe is clear (arrow).
	肺小型：肺全体が小さく、特に、左葉が顕著である（矢印）。

4-8　Absent lung lobe　　肺葉欠損　(New)

Species	Rabbit
Memo	Absent lung accessory lobe
	肺副葉欠損：肺副葉が欠損している。

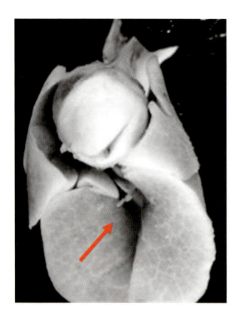
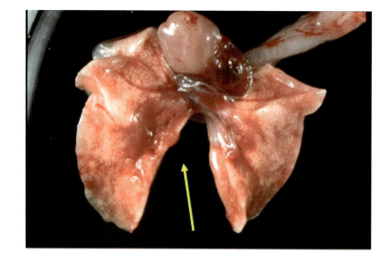

4-9   Fused lung lobe   肺葉癒合   (New)

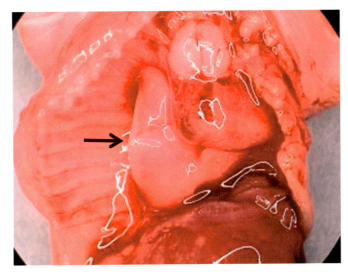

Species	Rabbit
Memo	Fused lung lobe, Non-separated lung lobe: The right lobe is one lobe without separating. It is also considered to be "Absent fissure of the lung lobe (New)".
	肺葉癒合、肺葉分離不全：右葉が分離していない。肺葉裂無形成（New）でも良い。

4-10 Supernumerary lobes of the lung   肺葉過剰   (10260)

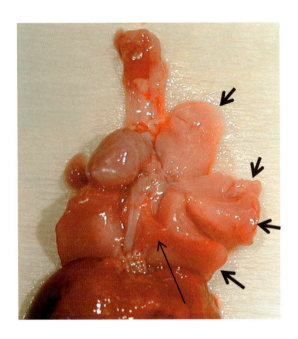

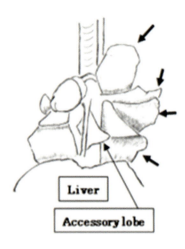

Species	Rabbit
Memo	Supernumerary lobes of the lung: 4 lobes at the left-side
	肺葉過剰：左葉が4葉

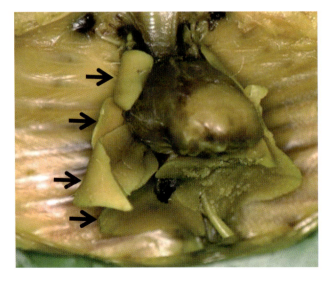

Species	Rat
Memo	Supernumerary lobes of the lung: 4 lobes at the right-side
	肺葉過剰：右葉が4葉

4-11 Diaphragmatic hernia　横隔膜ヘルニア　(10275)

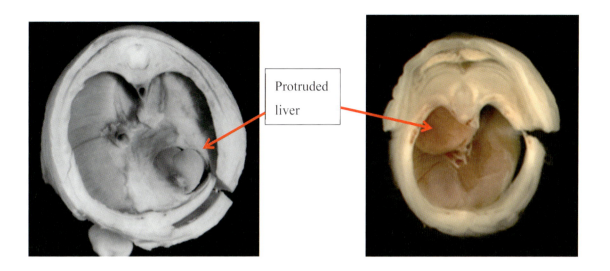

Species	Rat, Wistar
Memo	Diaphragmatic hernia: A part of the diaphragm is absent, and a part of the liver protrudes into the thorax.
	横隔膜ヘルニア：横隔膜の一部が欠損し、肝臓の一部が胸腔内に突出している。

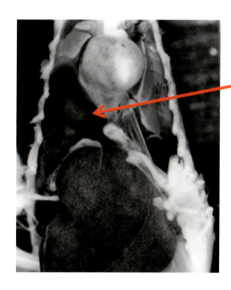

Species	Rabbit
Memo	Diaphragmatic hernia: Absence of portion of the diaphragm with protrusion of a part of the liver into the thorax.
	横隔膜ヘルニア：横隔膜の一部が欠損し、肝臓の一部が胸腔内に突出している。

4-11　Continued

Species	Rat, SD
Memo	Diaphragmatic hernia: A portion of the diaphragm is absent, and the intestine (left photo: red arrow) or a part of the liver (right photo: black arrow) protrudes into the thorax.
	横隔膜ヘルニア：横隔膜の一部が欠損し、腸管（左写真、赤矢印）あるいは肝臓の一部（右写真、黒矢印）が胸腔に突出している。

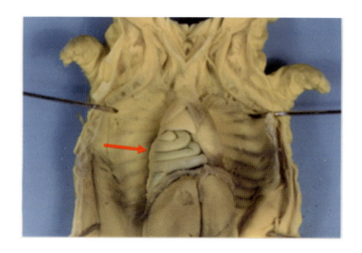
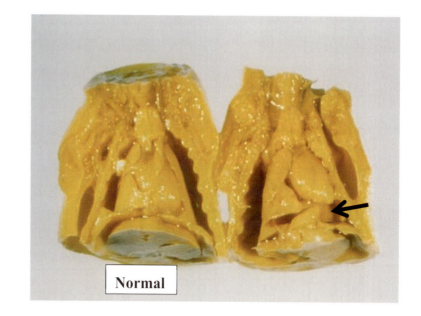

Photographs of Visceral Anomalies

5. Heart

5-1 Atrial septum defect 心房中隔欠損 (10171)

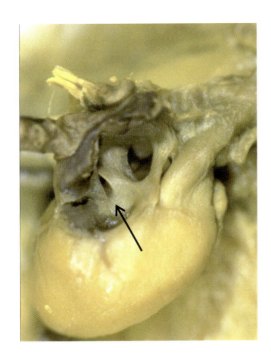

Species	Rat
Memo	Atrial septum defect
	心房中隔欠損

5-2 Persistent atrioventricular (A-V) canal　共通房室口遺残　(10194)

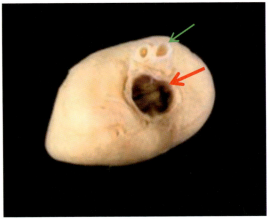

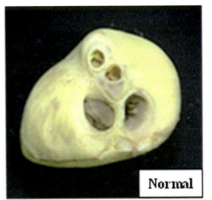
Normal

Species	Rat, SD
Memo	Persistent A-V canal (red arrow): Defects of endocardial cushions resulting in low atrial and high ventricular septal defects. Malpositioned aorta origin (New, green arrow) is also observed in this fetus. In internal observation of the ventricle, double outlet from the same (right) ventricle (New) is confirmed. A-V: atrioventricular
	共通房室口遺残（赤矢印）：心内膜クッションの欠損により心房中隔下部と心室中隔上部が欠損している。心房口が閉じずに残っている。大動脈起始部位置異常（New、緑矢印）も伴う。本例では、心室内部の観察で両大血管が右室から起始していること（両大血管起始：New）が確認されている。

Species	Rat
Memo	Persistent A-V canal (red arrow): Persistent truncus arteriosus (10223, black arrow) is also observed in this fetus.
	共通房室口遺残（赤矢印）：動脈幹遺残（10223、黒矢印）を伴う。

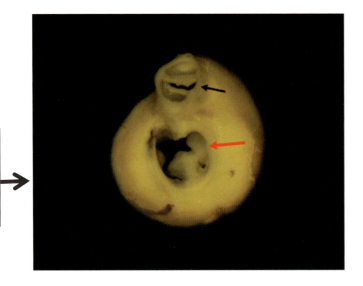

5-3 Premature closure of foramen ovale 卵円孔早期閉鎖 (New)

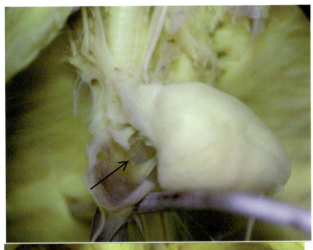

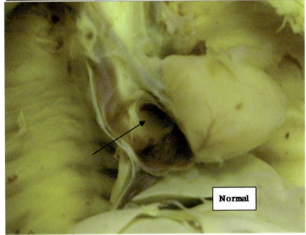

Species	Rat
Memo	Premature closure of foramen ovale: The foramen ovale is normally open in fetuses.
	卵円孔早期閉鎖：胎児期には通常開口している卵円孔が閉鎖している。

5-4　Misshapen heart　心臓形態異常　(New)

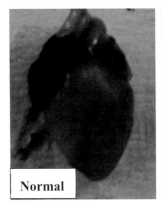 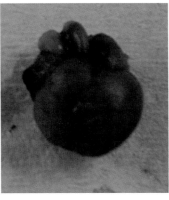

Species	Rabbit
Memo	Misshapen heart: Apex of the heart is not observed.
	心臓形態異常：心尖部が見られない。

5-5 Misshapen left atrioventricular (A-V) valve　左房室弁形態異常　(10190)

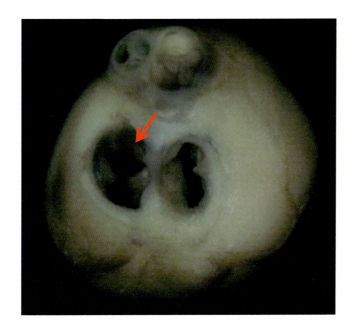

Species	Rat
Memo	Misshapen left A-V valve
	左房室弁形態異常

5-6 Misshapen pulmonary valve　肺動脈弁形態異常　(10191)

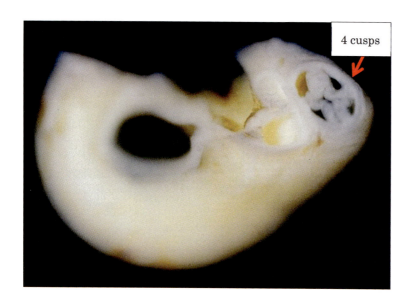

Species	Rat
Memo	Misshapen pulmonary valve: 4 cusps
	肺動脈弁形態異常：4尖弁

5-7 Double outlet from the right ventricle　両大血管起始（右室）　(New)

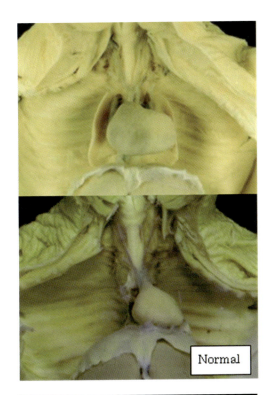

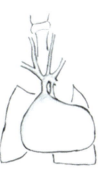

Normal

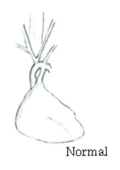

Normal

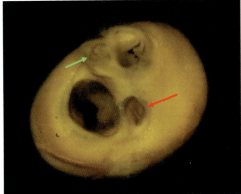

Species	Rat, SD
Memo	Double outlet from the right ventricle: Pulmonary trunk and aorta arise from the right ventricle. The right ventricle is large and the shape of the heart is abnormal. This fetus has "persistent A-V canal (10194)" and "Absent fissure of the right lobe of the lung (New)".
	両大血管起始（右室）：写真の方向から見た場合、通常、大動脈は肺動脈幹の後（背）方において左室より起始し、両大血管は螺旋状に（大動脈が肺動脈幹の前方に回りこみ）立ち上がるが、本標本では肺動脈幹の右側に相並んで（大動脈起始部位置異常：New）共に右室より起始し、両血管はほぼ並行して立ち上がっている。心外景は右室部が膨らんで心尖が目立たなくなり、やや扁平な形状を呈する（心臓形態異常：New）とともにやや大型化（10172）している。なお、本標本は共通房室口遺残（10194）及び肺の分葉異常（右葉裂無形成：New)を伴う。

Species	Rat
Memo	Double outlet from the right ventricle: The both of great arteries, aorta and pulmonary trunk, arise from the right ventricle. The right atrioventricular ostium (red arrow) and pulmonary trunk (10232, green arrow) are narrow.
	両大血管起始：右心室から大動脈及び肺動脈幹が起始している。右房室口（赤矢印）及び肺動脈幹（緑矢印）が細くなっている。

5-8 Ventricular septal defect 心室中隔欠損 (New)

Species	Rat
Memo	Membranous ventricular septum defect (VSD): An opening in the membranous septum between ventricles. In Ver.1, this code-No. is 10187 dividing from muscular VSD (10193).
	心室中隔膜性部欠損：心室中隔膜性部に孔が見られる。Ver.1 では 10187 とし、筋性部（10193）とは区分されている。

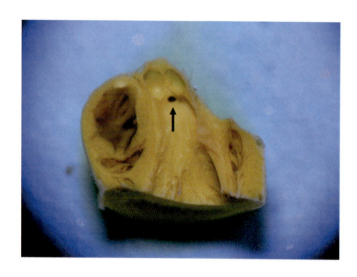

Rat, SD

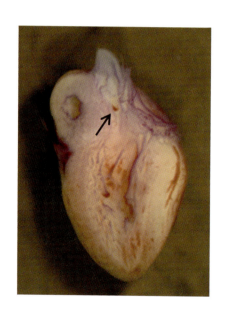

Rat, Wistar

5-9 Depression of ventricular septum 心室中隔陥没 (New)

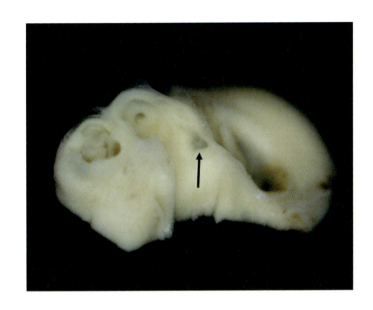

Species	Rat
Memo	Depression of ventricular septum: The membranous septum is thin and localized recess to the right ventricle is observed (arrow).
	心室中隔陥没：心室中隔膜性部が薄く、右心室側に陥没している（矢印）。

Photographs of Visceral Anomalies

6. Vessel

6. Abnormalities in the cardiovascular system　心・脈管系異常

For the structure of the heart, various abnormalities in the position of the aorta origin/pulmonary trunk origin, and arteries arising from the aortic arch, can develop and cause severe effects on post-natal development. Therefore, it is important to consider their development process and the effects of the structural changes on blood circulation when judging and evaluating these findings.

1. Structure of the Heart and Position of the Aorta origin/Pulmonary trunk origin

　The heart (atria and ventricles) and aorta origin/pulmonary trunk origin are formed after formation of the cardiac loop and septum. In this Atlas, the following findings produced by the abnormal development process of the heart and great vessels are compiled as photographs with their associated explanations: Atrial septum defect (5-1); Persistent atrioventricular (A-V) canal (5-2); Double outlet from the right ventricle (5-7), Ventricular septal defect (5-8); Malpositioned aorta origin (6-1); Transposition great vessels (6-11); and Persistent truncus arteriosus (6-12). Among these findings, "Double outlet from the right ventricle", "Transposition great vessels" and "Persistent truncus arteriosus" result in cyanotic changes in humans. These anomalies often show changes in the positions of great vessel origins and the balance of the right and left ventricles. In such cases, observation of the whole animal should include consideration of the abnormal connection among these vessels and ventricles.

2. Aortic arch and arteries arising from the aortic arch

　The non-symmetric single aortic arch structure and surrounding arteries are formed through the processes of development, and loss, of the aortic arch arteries (6 pairs in total in the right and left sides), which connect the aortic sac located in the cranial primitive endocardial tube, and the dorsal aorta (primitive descending aorta). In this Atlas, the following changes are produced by an abnormal process of development of these organs/tissues: Interrupted aortic arch (6-2); Narrow aortic arch (6-3); Retroesophageal aortic arch (6-4), and Right-sided aortic arch (6-5). Changes that can be produced in the branching in the aortic arch include: Supernumerary branch from the aortic arch (6-6); Malpositioned carotid origin (6-8); Long innominate artery (6-13); Supernumerary branch from the innominate artery (6-14); Malpositioned subclavian artery (6-17); Retroesophageal right subclavian artery (6-18); Supernumerary right subclavian artery (6-19); and Malpositioned subclavian artery origin (6-20). For the development of the aortic arch and great arteries, malformations that are produced by improper exchange of the blood vessels that should be deleted with those that should remain, "Retroesophageal aortic arch", "Right-sided aortic arch", "Malpositioned subclavian artery" and "Retroesophageal right subclavian artery" are compiled in this Atlas. These changes are observed together with abnormalities in the position and ramification of branch blood vessels, and are considered to affect blood circulation. On the other hand, for the "Supernumerary branch from the aortic arch" and "Supernumerary right subclavian artery" that are thought to be remnants of the blood vessels that should have resolved during the process of development, and for the "Malpositioned carotid origin", "Long innominate artery" and "Malpositioned subclavian artery" that should have displacement already at the time of branchial artery formation, there should be no functional (hemodynamic) damage and are regarded as "Variations (minor anomalies)" or "Alteration within normal range" of the branches arising from the aortic arch in humans.

　心臓の構造と大動脈、肺動脈幹の起始開口部位置並びに大動脈弓から分岐する動脈については、これらの発生過程における障害によって様々な異常が発現し、且つ、生後発生に重篤な影響を及ぼす所見も少なくない。したがって、心・脈管系の所見判断並びに評価に際しては、発生過程及びその構造変化がもたらす血液循環への影響を考慮することが重要である。

1. 心臓の構造と大動脈、肺動脈幹の起始開口部位置
　　心臓の内腔（心房、心室）と大動脈、肺動脈幹の起始開口部位置は心ループの形成と中隔の完成を経て形成される。本アトラスでは、この発生過程の障害によって生じ得る所見として心房中隔欠損（5-1）、共通房室口（管）遺残（5-2）、両大血管起始（5-7）、心室中隔欠損（5-8）、大動脈起始部位置異常（6-1）、大血管転換（6-11）及び動脈幹遺残（6-12）が掲載集録されている。これらの所見の内、両大血管起始、大血管転換、動脈幹遺残はヒトにおいてはチアノーゼ性の疾患とされる所見である。なお、両大血管起始、大血管転換では外景上に大動脈と肺動脈幹の起始部の位置関係及び左右心室のバランスの変化を認めることが多く、その様な場合には両血管と心室とのつながりに留意して観察を行う。

2. 大動脈弓とこれより分岐する動脈

　大動脈弓とその周囲の血管については、原始心膜筒の頭方に位置する大動脈嚢と脊索腹側尾方に位置する背側大動脈（原始下行大動脈）との間をつなぐ左右 6 対の大動脈弓（鰓弓動脈）の発生と消失の過程を経て、最終的に非対称性の単一な弓構造とこれから分岐する血管が形成される。本アトラスでは、この発生過程の障害によって生じ得る大動脈の所見として大動脈弓離断（6-2）、大動脈弓狭窄（6-3）、食道背方大動脈弓（6-4）、右側大動脈弓（6-5）、また、大動脈弓からの分岐に関する所見として大動脈弓過剰起始（6-6）、頸動脈起始部位置異常（6-8）、腕頭動脈伸長（6-13）、腕頭動脈過剰起始（6-14）、鎖骨下動脈位置異常（6-17）、食道背方鎖骨下動脈(6-18)、過剰鎖骨下動脈（6-19）及び鎖骨下動脈起始部位置異常（6-20）が掲載集録されている。大動脈弓分岐についてはさらに発生過程で消失すべき血管と残存すべき血管が入れ替わったと考えられる所見として食道背方大動脈弓、右側大動脈弓、鎖骨下動脈位置異常、食道背方鎖骨下動脈が挙げられ、これらの所見では何れも分岐血管の位置並びに走行に異常が認められる。一方、発生過程で消失すべき血管の残存と考えられる大動脈弓過剰起始、過剰鎖骨下動脈あるいは既に鰓弓動脈形成時の分岐に変位が生じていた可能性のある頸動脈起始部位置異常、腕頭動脈伸長、鎖骨下動脈起始部位置異常は何れも機能的（血行動態）な障害は無いと考えられ、ヒトでは大動脈弓分岐破格（Variation あるいは正常範囲内の変化）とされる所見である。

6-1 Malpositioned aorta origin　大動脈起始部位置異常　(New)

Species	Rat
Memo	Malpositioned aorta origin: The aorta origin (outlet from the heart) is dilated and displaced to outside comparing with normal fetus (arrow). Because the shape of the heart, balance of right and left ventricles, is abnormal, the observation of the internal in the heart and of passage between ventricles and aorta and pulmonary trunk should be done carefully. This fetus may be considered to have Double outlet from the right ventricle (New, see 5-7).
	大動脈起始部位置異常：大動脈起始部の拡張がみられ、正常に比べ外側（右側方向）に変位している（矢印）。心臓の形態（右心室と左心室のバランス）も異常で、心臓内部及び心室と両動脈とのつながりに注意して観察する必要がある。本例は両大血管起始（New、5-7 参照）と考えられる。

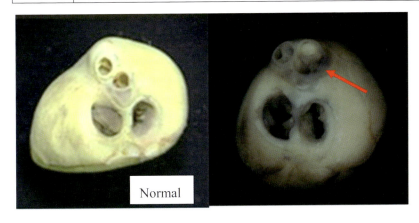

Normal

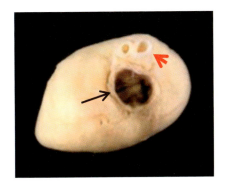

Species	Rat, SD
Memo	Malpositioned aorta origin (red arrow): Persistent A-V canal (black arrow, 10194) is also observed in this fetus. In internal observation of the ventricle, this is considered to be "Double outlet from same ventricle (New, see 5-7)".　　　　A-V: atrioventricular
	大動脈起始部位置異常：共通房室口遺残（10194）を伴う。本例では、心室内部の観察で両大血管が右室から起始していること（両大血管起始：New、5-7 参照）が確認されている。

6-2 Interrupted aortic arch　大動脈弓離断　(10208)

Species	Rat, SD
Memo	Interrupted aortic arch with Malpositioned right subclavian artery origin (New): A part of the aortic arch is absent, and the ascending aorta does not connect to the descending aorta. Both the carotid arteries and right subclavian artery arise from the ascending aorta, and left subclavian artery arises from the descending aorta. Confirm that the aortic arch is not passing behind the trachea and/or esophagus, because "Interrupted aortic arch" is similar to "Retroesophageal aortic arch" when observing from the ventral side.
	大動脈弓離断：上行大動脈と下行大動脈がつながらず、大動脈弓の一部が欠損している。左右総頸動脈と右鎖骨下動脈は上行大動脈から分岐しているが、左鎖骨下動脈は下行大動脈から分岐している。右鎖骨下動脈起始部位置異常（New）を伴う。腹側からの観察では「食道背方大動脈弓、Code No. 10210」と類似しているので、観察時には注意する。

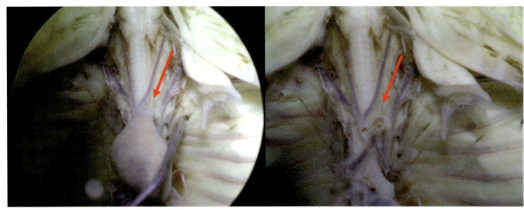

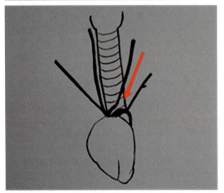

6-2 Continued

Species	Rabbit
Memo	Interrupted aortic arch: A part of the aortic arch is absent, and the ascending aorta does not connect to the descending aorta. Both the carotid arteries and right subclavian artery arise from the ascending aorta, and left subclavian artery arises from the descending aorta.
	大動脈弓離断：上行大動脈と下行大動脈がつながらず、大動脈弓の一部が欠損している。左右総頸動脈と右鎖骨下動脈は上行大動脈から分岐しているが、左鎖骨下動脈は下行大動脈から分岐している。

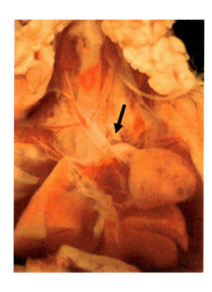
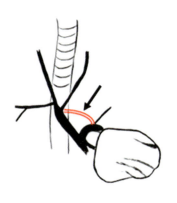
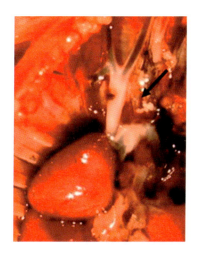
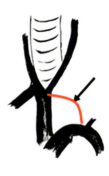

6-2 Continued

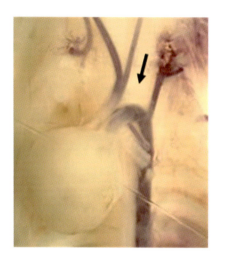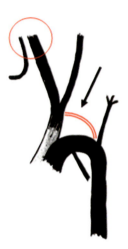

Species	Rat
Memo	Interrupted aortic arch with Long innominate artery (10226, red-circle in Fig): A part of the aortic arch is absent, and the ascending aorta does not connect to the descending aorta. Both the carotid arteries and right subclavian artery arise from the ascending aorta, and left subclavian artery arises from the descending aorta.
	大動脈弓離断：上行大動脈と下行大動脈がつながらず、大動脈弓の一部が欠損している。左右総頸動脈と右鎖骨下動脈は上行大動脈から分岐しているが、左鎖骨下動脈は下行大動脈から分岐している。腕頭動脈伸長（10226、図中の○）を伴う。

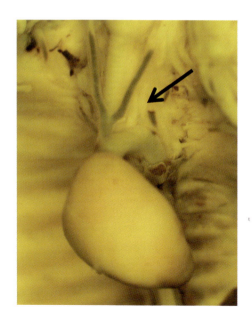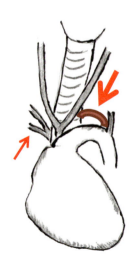

Species	Rat
Memo	Interrupted aortic arch (thick arrow in Fig.) with Retroesophageal right subclavian artery (10240, thin arrow in Fig.): A part of the aortic arch is absent, and the ascending aorta does not connect to the descending aorta. Both the carotid arteries arise from the ascending aorta, and left subclavian artery arises from the descending aorta.
	大動脈弓離断：上行大動脈と下行大動脈がつながらず、大動脈弓の一部が欠損している。左右総頸動脈は上行大動脈から分岐しているが、左鎖骨下動脈は下行大動脈から分岐している。食道背方右鎖骨下動脈（10240、図中の細矢印）を伴う。

6-2 Continued

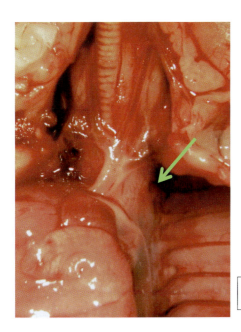
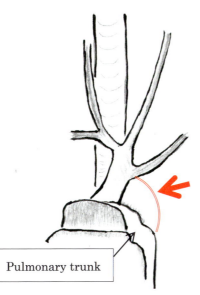

Pulmonary trunk

Species	Rabbit
Memo	Interrupted aortic arch: A part of the aortic arch is absent, and the ascending aorta does not connect to the descending aorta.
	大動脈弓離断：上行大動脈と下行大動脈がつながらず、大動脈弓の一部が欠損している。

6-3 Narrow aortic arch 大動脈弓狭窄 (10209)

Species	Rabbit
Memo	Narrow aortic arch: The aortic arch is generally narrow, and the pulmonary trunk and the ductus arteriosus are dilated (10231 and 10218, respectively).
	大動脈弓狭窄：上行大動脈及び大動脈弓が狭窄しており、肺動脈幹及び動脈管が拡張している（10231及び10218）。

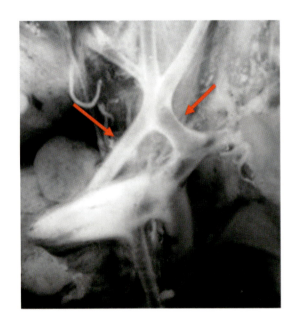
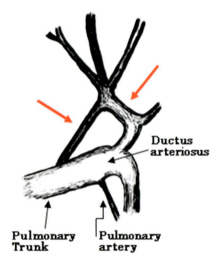

6-3 Continued

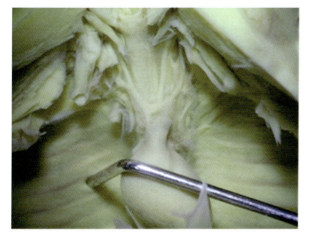

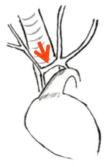

Species	Rat
Memo	Narrow aortic arch with Dilated pulmonary trunk (10231): The aortic arch is narrow and the pulmonary trunk is dilated. Although ventricular septum defect (New) is observed, no abnormalities are observed in both ventricles in this fetus.
	大動脈弓狭窄：上行大動脈及び大動脈弓が狭窄し、肺動脈幹が拡張（10231）している。本胎児では、心室中隔欠損（New）も認められ、大動脈への心排出口も狭小化しているが、心室には顕著な異常は認められていない。

Species	Rat
Memo	Narrow aortic arch with Malpositioned subclavian artery origin (New): The aortic arch is narrow between the left carotid artery origin and ductus arteriosus outlet.
	大動脈弓狭窄：大動脈弓が左頸動脈起始部から動脈管開口部の間で狭窄している。右鎖骨下動脈起始部位置異常（New）を伴う。

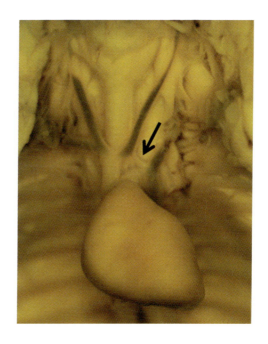
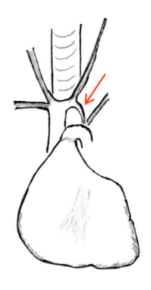

6-3 Continued

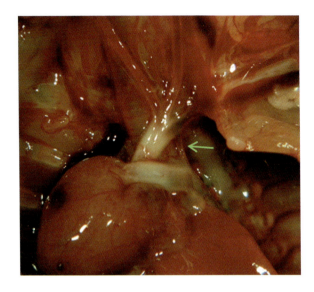
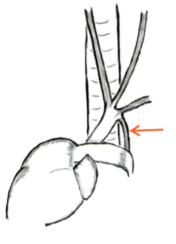

Species	Rabbit
Memo	Narrow aortic arch: The aortic arch is narrow between the left subclavian artery origin and ductus arteriosus outlet. The right subclavian artery is not clearly visible in this photograph.
	大動脈弓狭窄：大動脈弓が左鎖骨下動脈起始部から動脈管開口部の間で狭窄している。本写真では右鎖骨下動脈が不明。

6-4　Retroesophageal aortic arch　食道背方大動脈弓　(10210)

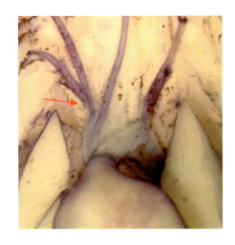 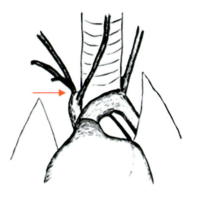

Species	Rat
Memo	Retroesophageal aortic arch with Malpositioned right subclavian artery origin (New, red arrow in Fig): The aortic arch passes behind the esophagus and trachea.
	食道背方大動脈弓：大動脈弓が食道及び気管の背側を走行し、血管輪を形成している。右鎖骨下動脈起始部位置異常（New、図中の矢印）を伴う。

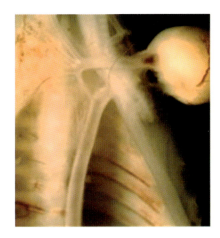 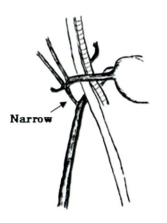

Species	Rat
Memo	Retroesophageal aortic arch: The aortic arch is narrow and passes behind the esophagus and trachea.
	食道背方大動脈弓：大動脈弓が細く、食道及び気管の背側を走行し、血管輪を形成している。

6-4 Continued

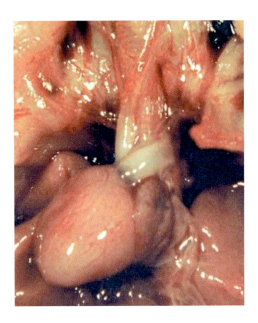

Species	Rabbit
Memo	Retroesophageal aortic arch: The aortic arch passes behind the esophagus and trachea.
	食道背方大動脈弓：大動脈弓が食道及び気管の背側を走行し、血管輪を形成している。

6-5 Right-sided aortic arch　　右側大動脈弓　(10211)

Species	Rabbit
Memo	Right-sided aortic arch
	右側大動脈弓

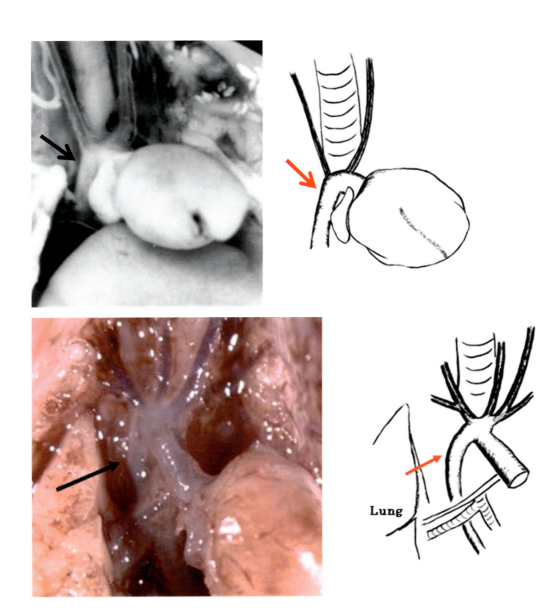

6-5 Continued

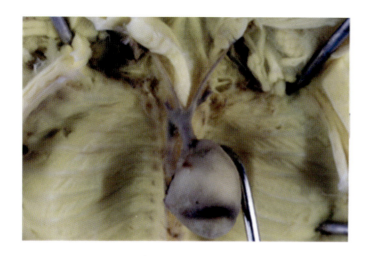

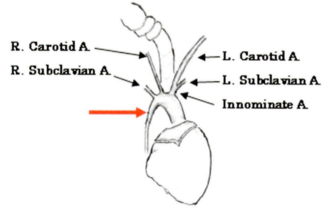

Species	Rat, SD
Memo	Right-sided aortic arch: The left subclavian and left carotid arteries arise from the innominate artery which arises at the left-side of the aortic arch. The right carotid and right subclavian arteries arise directly from the aortic arch following the innominate artery.
	右側大動脈弓：大動脈弓が右側へ走行している。大動脈弓からの血管分岐は、先ず腕頭動脈が起始し、これより左鎖骨下動脈及び左総頸動脈が分岐し、次に右総頸動脈、右鎖骨下動脈の順に起始しており、正常に対して鏡像を示す。

6-6 Supernumerary branch from the aortic arch   大動脈弓過剰起始   (New)

Species	Rabbit
Memo	Supernumerary branch from the aortic arch with Supernumerary branch from the innominate artery: Additional arteries (A), which may be internal thoracic artery, subscapular artery or vertebral artery, arise directly from the aortic arch. In rabbits, this type of anomaly is occasionally observed, so it may be considered within normal range. In a survey of companies, half described this alternation in rabbits as a "malformation" while the other half described it as "normal". The internal carotid artery (B) arises from the innominate artery.
	大動脈弓過剰起始：付加的な動脈（図A：内胸動脈、肩甲下動脈あるいは椎骨動脈）が大動脈弓左側から直接分岐している。ウサギではまま見られるものであり、所見としない場合もある。複数の施設での採用状況を確認したところ、半数の施設では「異常」として、半数の施設では「正常範囲内の変化（正常）」としている。内頸動脈（図B）が腕頭動脈から分岐している（New：腕頭動脈過剰起始）。

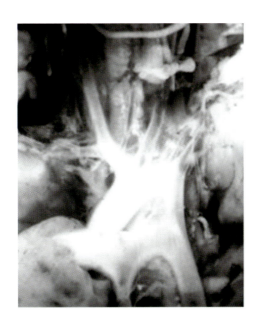
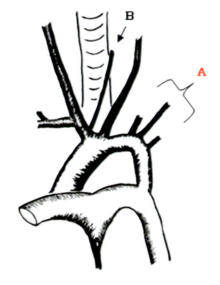

6-6 Continued

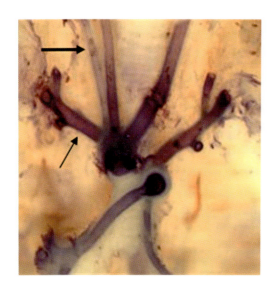 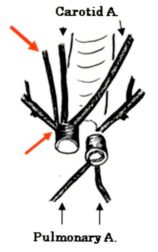

Species	Rat
Memo	Supernumerary branch from the aortic arch with Malpositioned subclavian artery origin (New): An additional artery (thick arrow) arises from the aortic arch, and the right subclavian artery (thin arrow) arises directly from the aortic arch (New).
	大動脈弓過剰起始：付加的な動脈が大動脈弓から起始している。鎖骨下動脈起始部位置異常（右鎖骨下動脈が大動脈弓から直接起始している。New）を伴う。

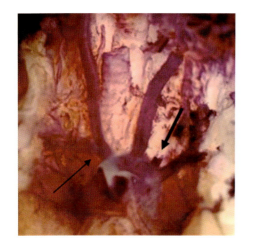 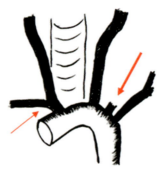

Species	Rat
Memo	Supernumerary branch from the aortic arch: An additional artery (thick arrow), which may be subscapular artery, arises directly from the aortic arch. The right subclavian artery (thin arrow) arises from lower point of the innominate artery (Malpositioned subclavian artery origin: New, or, Short innominate artery: 10229).
	大動脈弓過剰起始：付加的な動脈（おそらく肩甲下動脈）が大動脈弓から直接起始している。右鎖骨下動脈起始部位置異常（大動脈弓近位の腕頭動脈から起始している：New、あるいは、腕頭動脈短小：10229）を伴う。

6-6 Continued

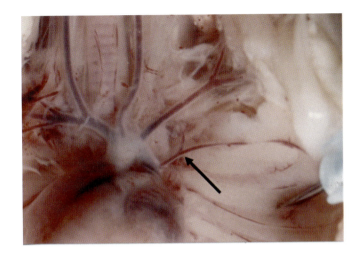

Species	Rabbit
Memo	Supernumerary artery from the aortic arch: Additional artery (maybe vertebral artery) arises directly from the aortic arch.
	大動脈弓過剰起始：付加的動脈（椎骨動脈）が直接大動脈弓から分岐している。

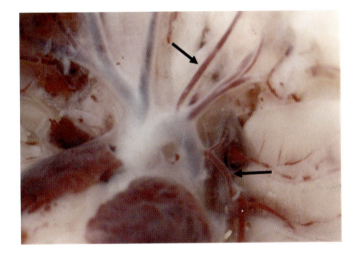

Species	Rabbit
Memo	Supernumerary artery from the aortic arch: Additional arteries (maybe internal thoracic artery, vertebral artery, or subscapular artery) arise directly from the aortic arch.
	大動脈弓過剰起始：付加的動脈（内胸動脈、椎骨動脈、あるいは肩甲下動脈）が直接大動脈弓から分岐している。

6-6 Continued

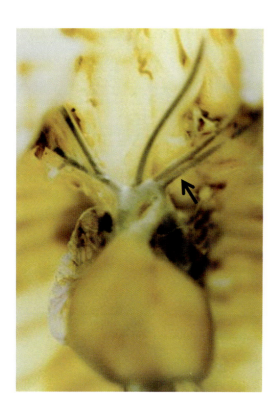

Species	Rat
Memo	Supernumerary artery from the aortic arch: Additional arteries (maybe internal thoracic artery, vertebral artery, or subscapular artery) arise directly from the aortic arch.
	大動脈弓過剰起始：付加的動脈（内胸動脈、椎骨動脈、あるいは肩甲下動脈）が直接大動脈弓から分岐している。

6-7 Supernumerary artery   動脈過剰   (New)

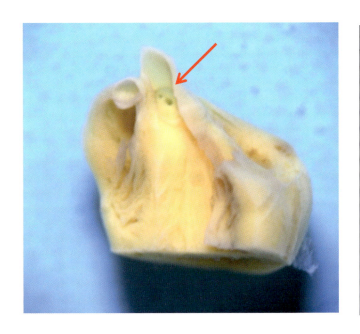

Species	Rat, SD
Memo	Supernumerary artery: Supernumerary right coronary arteries which directly arise from the aorta. In rats and rabbits, the number of right coronary ostium at the aorta is one in normal fetuses, however, fetuses with 2 ostia or more were sometimes observed as shown in these photographs. Although "Supernumerary right coronary ostium" is better term, this name is used because the term "Supernumerary right coronary ostium" is not in the harmonized terminology of the developmental anomalies.
	動脈過剰：大動脈から直接分岐している右冠状動脈が多い。通常分岐（右冠状動脈口）は1個で、ラットやウサギでは本例の様に2個あるいはそれ以上の場合がある。「右冠状動脈口過剰」と言う所見が妥当であり、統一用語には「右冠状動脈口過剰」がないので、ここに掲載する。

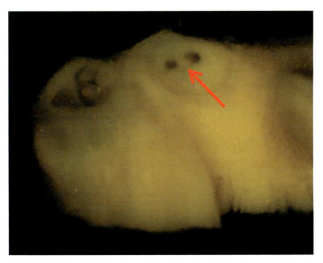
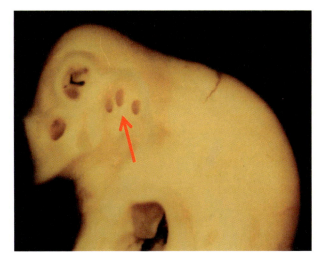

6-8 Malpositioned carotid origin   頸動脈起始部位置異常   (New)

Species	Rat
Memo	Malpositioned carotid origin: The left carotid artery arises near the innominate artery (thick arrow). The right subclavian artery arises near the junction of the innominate artery (thin arrow, Malpositioned subclavian artery origin: New, or, Short innominate artery: 10229).
	頸動脈起始部位置異常：左頸動脈が腕頭動脈付近で分岐している。右鎖骨下動脈起始部位置異常（大動脈弓近位の腕頭動脈から起始している、New）、あるいは、腕頭動脈短小（10229）を伴う。

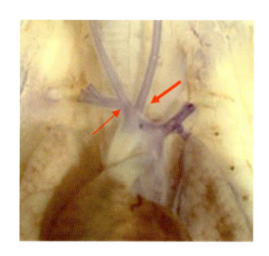
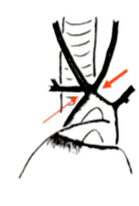

6-8 Continued

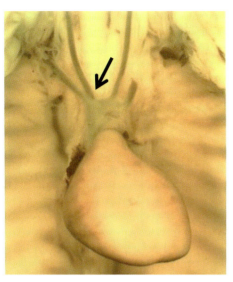

Species	Rat
Memo	Malpositioned carotid origin: The right carotid artery arises from the aortic arch.
	頸動脈起始部位置異常：右頸動脈が直接大動脈弓から起始している。

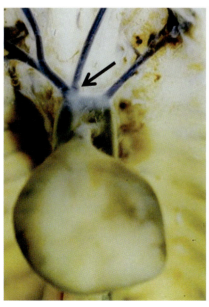

Species	Rat
Memo	Malpositioned carotid origin: The left carotid artery arises near the innominate artery.
	頸動脈起始部位置異常：左頸動脈が腕頭動脈付近で分岐している。

6-9 Dilated ductus arteriosus　　動脈管拡張（化）　（10218）

Species	Rabbit
Memo	Dilated ductus arteriosus: The ductus arteriosus is dilated as well as the pulmonary trunk (10231) resulting in a generally narrow aortic arch (10209).
	動脈管拡張（化）：大動脈弓全体が狭窄しており（10209）、その影響で、肺動脈幹拡張（10231）と共に動脈管が拡張している。

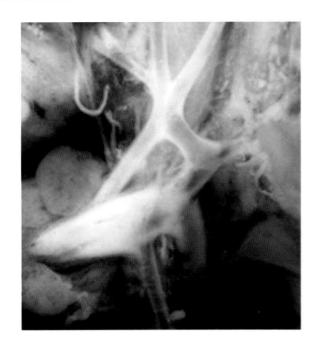
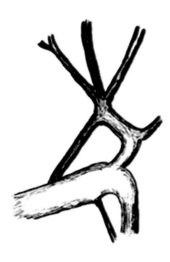

6-10　Narrow ductus arteriosus　　動脈管狭窄　（10220)

Species	Rabbit
Memo	Narrow ductus arteriosus (arrow) with Malpositioned left carotid origin (New) and Supernumerary branch from the aortic arch (New)
	動脈管狭窄：左頸動脈起始部位置異常（New）及び大動脈弓過剰起始（New）を伴う。

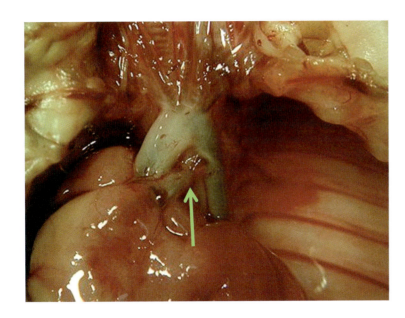
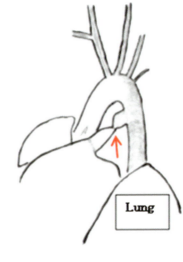

6-11 Transposition of great vessels 大血管転換 (10224)

Species	Rat
Memo	Transposition of great vessels: Origin of aorta from right ventricle and pulmonary trunk from left ventricle
	大血管転換：大動脈は右心室から、肺動脈幹は左心室から起始している。

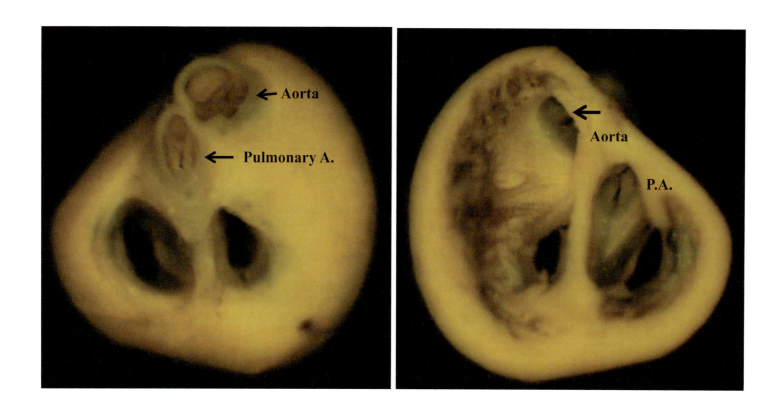

6-12　Persistent truncus arteriosus　動脈幹遺残　(10223)

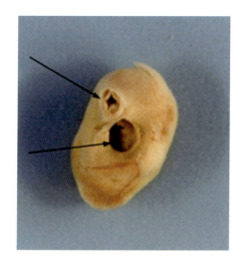

Species	Rat, SD
Memo	Persistent truncus arteriosus with Persistent A-V canal (10194)
	A-V: atrioventricular
	動脈幹遺残：動脈幹口から4個の半月弁が確認できる。共通房室口遺残（10194）を伴う。

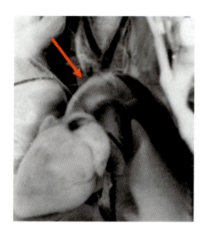 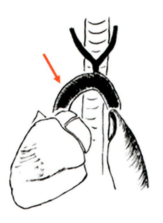

Species	Rabbit
Memo	Persistent truncus arteriosus
	動脈幹遺残：大動脈と肺動脈幹が1本になっている。

6-12 Continued

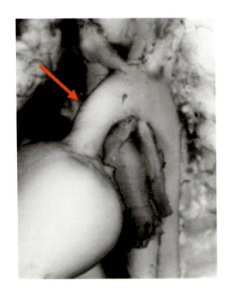
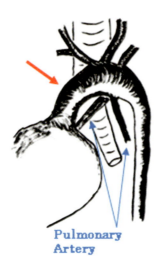

Species	Rabbit
Memo	Persistent truncus arteriosus
	動脈幹遺残：大動脈と肺動脈幹が分離せず、1本になっている。

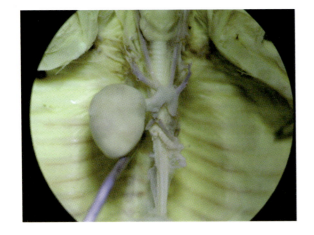

Species	Rat
Memo	Persistent truncus arteriosus: Aorta and pulmonary trunk are not divided. The carotid arteries, subclavian arteries and pulmonary arteries arise from this vessel. In this fetus, ventricular septum defect (VSD) was observed on the internal heart.
	動脈幹遺残：動脈幹が分割されず1本の血管として心臓と接続している。頸動脈、鎖骨下動脈及び肺動脈がこの血管から分岐している。本胎児では心臓内部の観察で心室中隔欠損（New）も見られている。

6-13 Long innominate artery 腕頭動脈伸長 (10226)

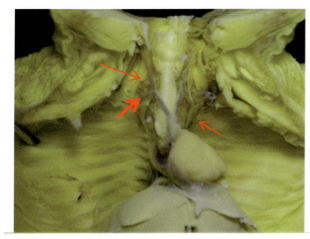

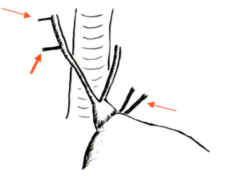

Species	Rat, SD
Memo	Long innominate artery with Supernumerary branch from the aortic arch (New): The right subclavian artery (thick arrow) arises from a distal point of the innominate artery. An additional artery (thin arrow), which may be the right subscapular artery, arises from the right carotid artery. Another artery, which may be the left vertebral artery, arises from the aortic arch similar to the left subclavian artery.
	腕頭動脈伸長：右鎖骨下動脈が正常より遠位で腕頭動脈（無名動脈）から分岐している。他の動脈（肩甲下動脈？）も総頸動脈から分岐している。大動脈弓過剰起始（New、左鎖骨下動脈と同様に他の動脈が直接大動脈弓から分岐している）もみられる。

6-14 Supernumerary branch from the innominate artery　　腕頭動脈過剰起始　(New)

Species	Rabbit
Memo	Supernumerary branch from the innominate artery with Supernumerary branch from the aortic arch (New): The internal carotid artery (A) arises from the innominate artery. Additional arteries (B), which may be internal thoracic artery, subscapular artery or vertebral artery, arise directly from the aortic arch. In rabbits, this type of anomaly is sometime observed, so it may be considered within normal range.
	腕頭動脈過剰起始：内頚動脈（図A）が腕頭動脈から直接分岐している。付加的な動脈（図B：内胸動脈、肩甲下動脈あるいは椎骨動脈）が大動脈弓左側から直接分岐している（New、大動脈弓過剰起始）。ウサギではまま見られるものであり、所見としない場合もある。

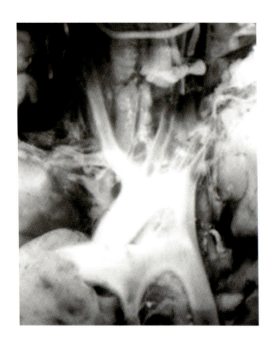 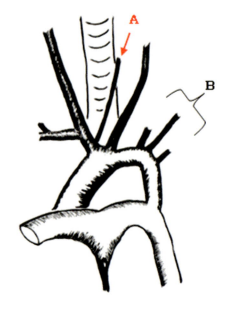

6-15 Dilated pulmonary trunk　　肺動脈幹拡張（化）　　(10231)

Species	Rabbit
Memo	Dilated pulmonary trunk: The pulmonary trunk is dilated as well as the ductus arteriosus (10218) leading to a generally narrowed aortic arch (10209).
	肺動脈幹拡張（化）：大動脈弓全体が狭窄しており（10209）、その影響で、動脈管拡張（10218）と共に肺動脈幹が拡張している。

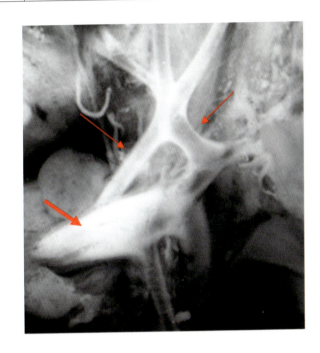
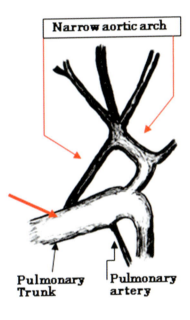

6-15 Continued

Species	Rat
Memo	Dilated pulmonary trunk with Narrow aortic arch (10209): The aortic arch is narrow, and pulmonary trunk is dilated. Ventricular septum defect (New) is generally observed, however, no abnormalities were observed in both ventricles in this fetus.
	肺動脈幹拡張：大動脈弓が狭窄（10209）し、肺動脈幹が拡張している。本胎児では、心室中隔欠損（New）も認められ、大動脈への心排出口も狭小化しているが、心室には顕著な異常は認められていない。

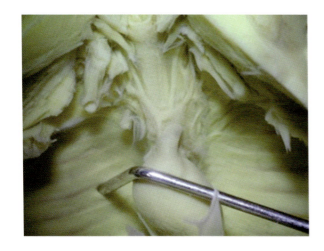 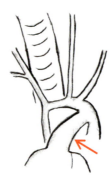

6-16 Narrow pulmonary trunk　肺動脈幹狭窄　(10232)

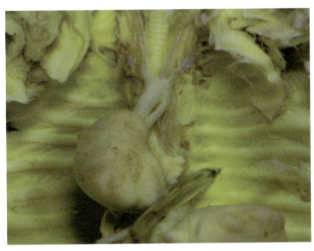

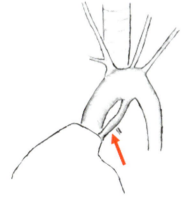

Species	Rat
Memo	Narrow pulmonary trunk: The outlet from the heart displaces to right-side. This is considered to be tetralogy of Fallot because this fetus has narrow pulmonary trunk, VSD (New), and overriding aorta (10205). This fetus also has large right ventricular chamber (10183) and thick right ventricular wall (10184).
	肺動脈幹狭窄：大動脈起始部位置異常（New：心排出口の右側への変位）に加え、心室中隔欠損（New）、大動脈の騎乗（10205）、右心室腔の拡張（10183）及び壁肥厚（10184)が認められ、Fallot四徴症と診断された。

6-17 Malpositioned subclavian artery 鎖骨下動脈位置異常 (10238)

Species	Rabbit
Memo	Malpositioned subclavian artery: The right subclavian artery arises at the dorsal site of the aortic arch and passes in front of the trachea. May also be judged as "Malpositioned subclavian artery origin (New)".
	鎖骨下動脈位置異常：右鎖骨下動脈が大動脈弓の背側から分岐し、気管の腹側を走行している。鎖骨下動脈起始部位置異常（New）でも良い。

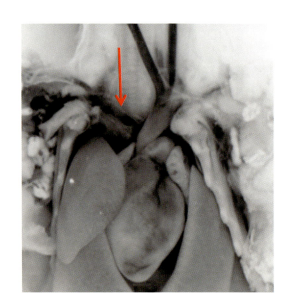
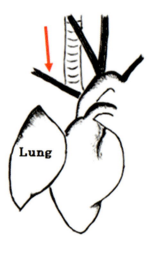

6-18 Retroesophageal right subclavian artery   食道背方右鎖骨下動脈 (10240)

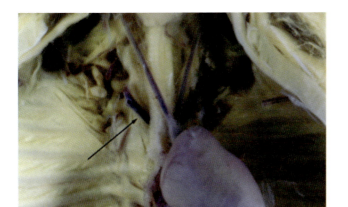

Species	Rat
Memo	Retroesophageal right subclavian artery: The right subclavian artery passes behind the esophagus. Usually, this artery originates at dorsal position of the aortic arch, and passes behind the trachea and esophagus.
	食道背方右鎖骨下動脈：右鎖骨下動脈が食道の背方を走行している。多くの場合、大動脈弓の背側から起始し、気管及び食道の背方を走行している。

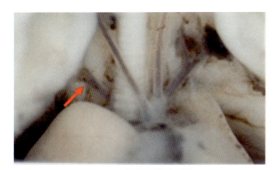
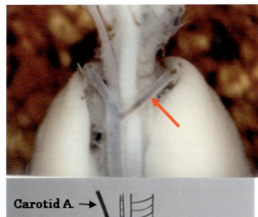
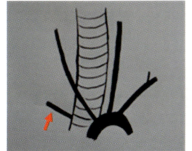
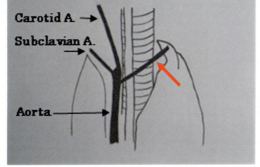

6-18 Continued

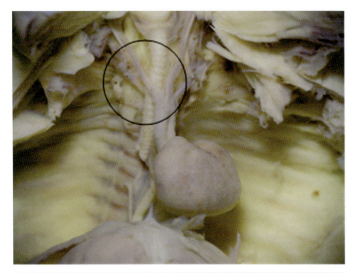

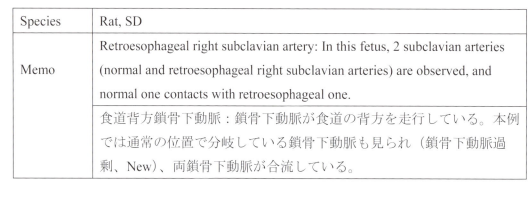

Species	Rat, SD
Memo	Retroesophageal right subclavian artery: In this fetus, 2 subclavian arteries (normal and retroesophageal right subclavian arteries) are observed, and normal one contacts with retroesophageal one.
	食道背方鎖骨下動脈：鎖骨下動脈が食道の背方を走行している。本例では通常の位置で分岐している鎖骨下動脈も見られ（鎖骨下動脈過剰、New）、両鎖骨下動脈が合流している。

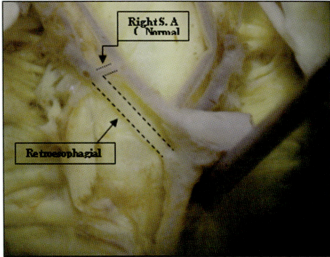

6-18 Continued

Species	Rabbit
Memo	Retroesophageal right subclavian artery: The right subclavian artery arises at dorsal position of the aortic arch and passes behind the trachea and esophagus.
	食道背方右鎖骨下動脈：右鎖骨下動脈が大動脈弓の背側で起始し、気管及び食道の背側を走行している。

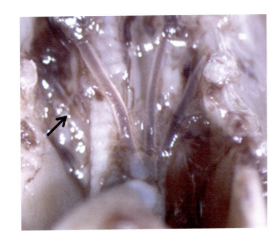
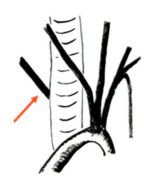

6-19 Supernumerary subclavian artery　鎖骨下動脈過剰　(New)

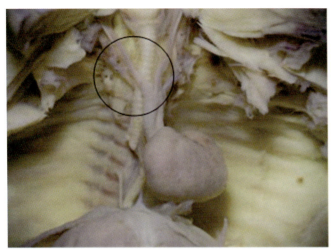

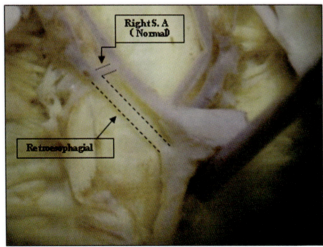

Species	Rat, SD
Memo	Supernumerary right subclavian artery: In this fetus, 2 subclavian arteries (normal and retroesophageal right subclavian arteries) are observed, and normal one contacts with retroesophageal one.
	右鎖骨下動脈過剰：食道の背方を走行している鎖骨下動脈（食道背方鎖骨下動脈、10240）と通常の位置で分岐している鎖骨下動脈の2本の鎖骨下動脈が見られ、両鎖骨下動脈が合流している。

6-20 Malpositioned subclavian artery origin 鎖骨下動脈起始部位置異常 (New)

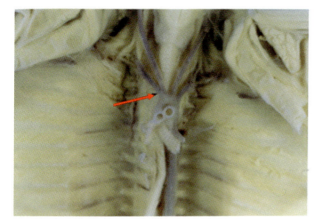

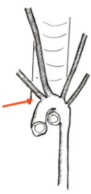

Species	Rat
Memo	Malpositioned right subclavian artery origin: The right subclavian artery arises directly from the aortic arch, and the innominate artery is absent.
	鎖骨下動脈起始部位置異常：右鎖骨下動脈が大動脈弓から直接分岐し、腕頭動脈が見られない。

6-20 Continued

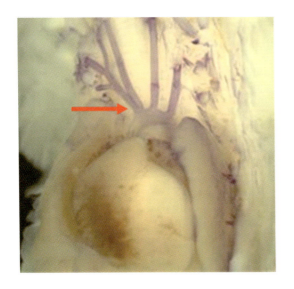
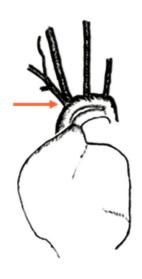

Species	Rat
Memo	Malpositioned subclavian artery origin: The right subclavian artery arises directly from the aortic arch.
	鎖骨下動脈起始部位置異常：右鎖骨下動脈が大動脈弓から直接分岐している。

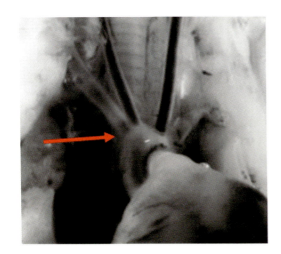
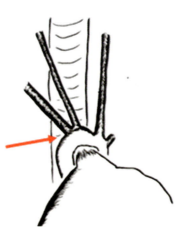

Species	Rat
Memo	Malpositioned subclavian artery origin: The right subclavian artery arises directly from the aortic arch.
	鎖骨下動脈起始部位置異常：右鎖骨下動脈が大動脈弓から直接分岐している。

6-20 Continued

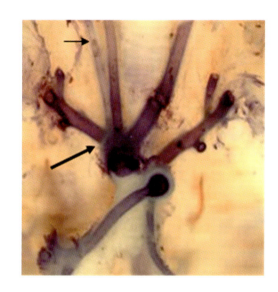
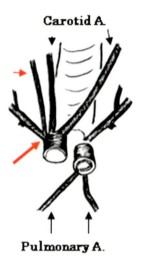

Species	Rat
Memo	Malpositioned subclavian artery origin (thick arrow) with Supernumerary branch from the aortic arch (thin arrow, New): The right subclavian artery arises directly from the aortic arch, and an additional artery also arises from the aortic arch.
	鎖骨下動脈起始部位置異常（太矢印）：右鎖骨下動脈が大動脈弓から起始している。付加的な動脈が大動脈弓から起始している（細矢印、大動脈弓過剰起始、New）。

6-21 Bilateral umbilical artery 両側臍動脈 (New)

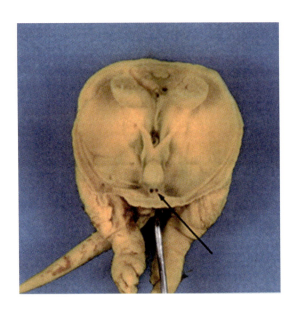

Species	Rat, SD
Memo	Bilateral umbilical artery: In this fetus, 2 umbilical arteries pass at the abdominal side of the urinary bladder although 1 umbilical artery normally passes at the right-side of the urinary bladder.
	両側臍動脈：ラットでは、臍動脈は1本で膀胱の右側を走行するが、本例では、膀胱の腹側を2本走行している。

6-22　Transposed umbilical artery　臍動脈転換　(New)

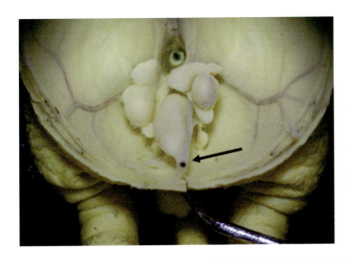

Species	Rat, SD
Memo	Transposed umbilical artery, or Left umbilical artery: In rats, umbilical artery usually passes at the right-side of the urinary bladder, however, this artery passes to the left-side in this fetus.
	臍動脈転換：左臍動脈、あるいは、臍動脈左側存在とも言う。ラットの場合臍動脈は膀胱の右側を走行するが、本例は膀胱の左側を走行している。

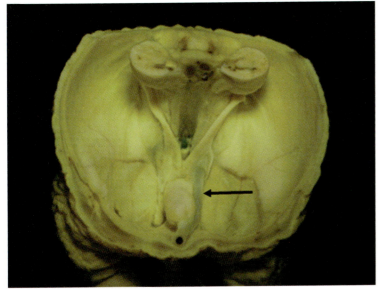

Species	Rat
Memo	Transposed umbilical artery, or Left umbilical artery: In rats, umbilical artery usually passes at the right-side of the urinary bladder, however, this artery passes to the left-side in this fetus.
	臍動脈転換：左臍動脈、あるいは、臍動脈左側存在とも言う。ラットの場合臍動脈は膀胱の右側を走行するが、本例は膀胱の左側を走行している。

6-23　Bilateral azygos veins　両側奇静脈　(10272)

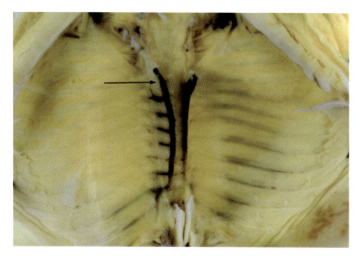

Species	Rat, SD
Memo	Bilateral azygos veins, Supernumerary azygos veins, or Persistent right azygos vein: In rats, the azygos vein is observed only at the left side of the spine. In this fetus, the azygos veins are observed bilaterally.
	両側奇静脈：ラットでは、奇静脈は脊柱の左側のみを走行するが、本例では両側を走行している。

6-24 Transposed azygos vein   奇静脈転換   (10273)

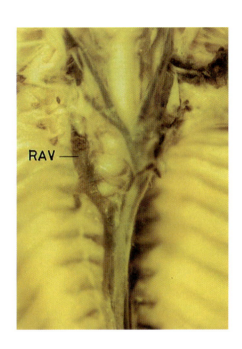

Species	Rat
Memo	Transposed azygos vein: Azygos vein passes at the right-side (RAV).
	奇静脈転換：奇静脈が右側を走行している。

6-25　Malpositioned posterior (caudal) vena cava　　後（尾側）大静脈位置異常　(10269)

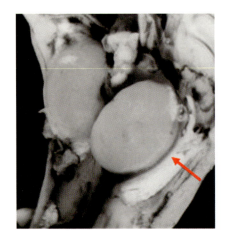 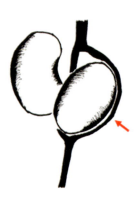

Species	Rabbit
Memo	Malpositioned posterior (caudal) vena cava: The vena cava is duplicated and passes at the side of the left kidney. This finding may also be referred to as "Branching variation of the posterior vena cava (New)".
	後（尾側）大静脈位置異常：後大静脈が分岐（重複）し、左腎臓の外側を走行している。後大静脈分岐変異（New）でも良い。

Photographs of Visceral Anomalies

7. Abdominal Organs

7-1 Misshapen liver　肝臓形態異常　(10284)

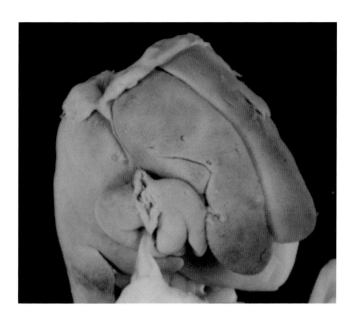

Species	Rabbit
Memo	Misshapen liver with Additional fissure of the liver (New): Abnormal shape of lobes and supernumerary lobes of the liver. This may be "Supernumerary lobes of the liver (10287)".
	肝臓形態異常：全体的に葉の形、数が異常。肝臓葉過剰（10287）でも良い。肝臓葉過剰形成裂（New）もみられる。

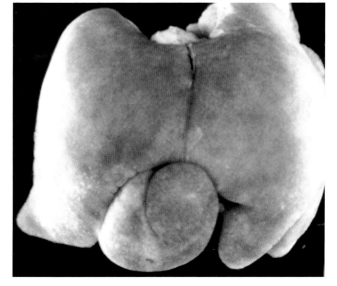

Species	Rabbit
Memo	Misshapen liver
	肝臓形態異常

7-2 Absent lobe of the liver　肝臓葉欠損　(New)

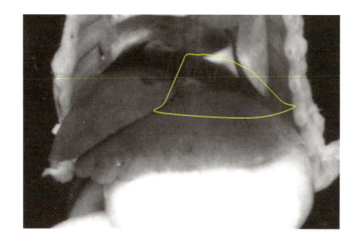

Species	Rabbit
Memo	Absent lobe of the liver: The left lateral lobe is absent.
	肝臓葉欠損：外側左葉が欠損している。

7-3 Additional fissures of the liver 肝臓葉過剰形成裂 (New)

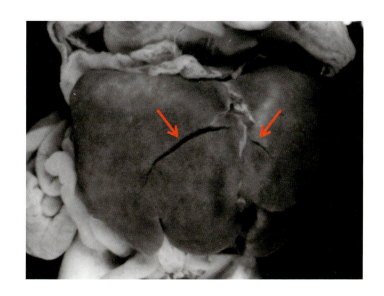

Species	Rabbit
Memo	Additional fissures of the liver: Additional fissures are observed in the right lateral lobe and left lateral lobe of the liver.
	肝臓葉過剰形成裂：外側右葉及び外側左葉に過剰な葉間裂が見られる。

7-4 Supernumerary lobes of the liver　肝臓葉過剰　(10287)

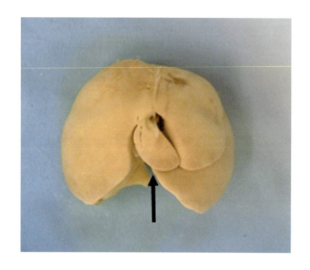

Species	Rat, SD
Memo	Supernumerary lobes of the liver
	肝臓葉過剰

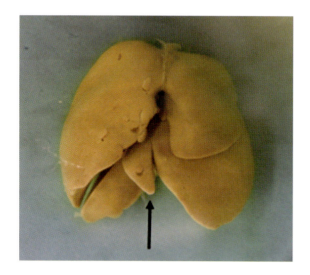

Species	Rat, SD
Memo	Supernumerary lobes of the liver: It is possible that this fetus has "Additional fissure of the liver lobe (New)", however, this case is routinely judged as "Supernumerary lobes" because the additional lobe is completely separated from the left medial lobe.
	肝臓葉過剰：肝臓葉過剰形成裂（Additional fissure, New）と言う所見も考えられるが、外観上、過剰な小葉が内側左葉から分離しており、実務上は「葉過剰」とするのが良いと考えられる。両所見については、判断に迷う例もあり、化合物の毒性を判断する場合には、複数の胎児の形態から統一した所見を選択することが望まれる。

7-5 Bilobed gallbladder 胆嚢二葉 (10290)

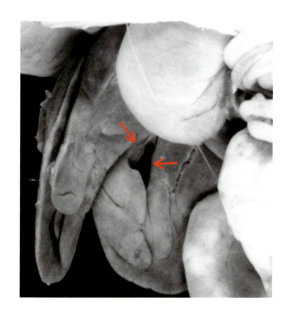

Species	Rabbit
Memo	Bilobed gallbladder: Duplicated gallbladders are observed.
	胆嚢二葉：胆嚢が重複している。

7-6 Supernumerary spleen 脾臓過剰 (10317)

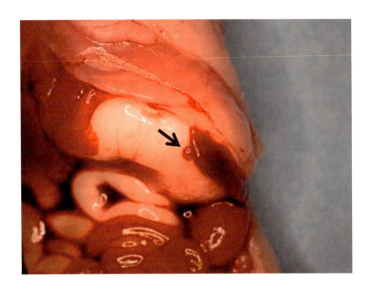

Species	Rabbit
Memo	Supernumerary spleen: Splenulus is observed.
	脾臓過剰：副脾がみられる。

7-7   **Absent intestine**   腸欠損   (10318)

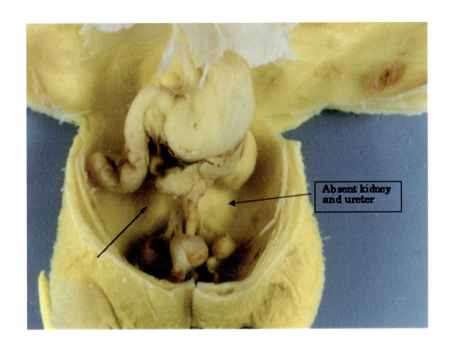

Species	Rat, SD
Memo	Absent intestine with Absent kidney (10326) and Absent ureter (10356)
	腸欠損：小腸及び大腸が欠損している。腎臓欠損(10326)及び尿管欠損(10356)を伴う。

7-8　Malpositioned intestine　腸位置異常　(10323)

Species	Rat, SD
Memo	Malpositioned intestine: The intestine protrudes into the subcutis through a hole in the peritoneum. This is a type of "Inguinal hernia".
	腸位置異常：右鼠径部腹壁欠損部より消化管が皮下に迷入している。ある種の鼠径ヘルニアである。

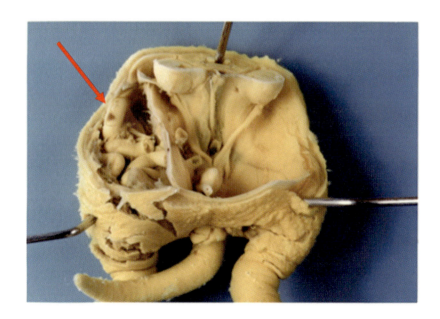
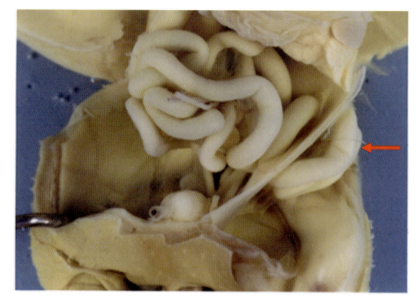

7-9 Absent kidney 腎臓欠損 (10326)

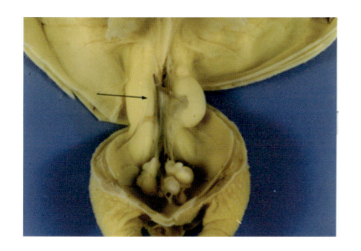

Species	Rat, SD
Memo	Absent kidney (right) with Absent adrenal (right, 10343) and Absent ureter (right, 10356)
	腎臓欠損：右腎臓が欠損している。副腎欠損（右 10343）及び尿管欠損（10356）を伴う。

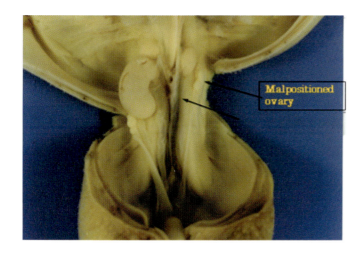

Species	Rat, SD
Memo	Absent kidney (left) with Malpositioned ovary (left, 10386)
	腎臓欠損：左腎臓が欠損している。卵巣位置異常（左 10386）を伴う。

7-9 Continued

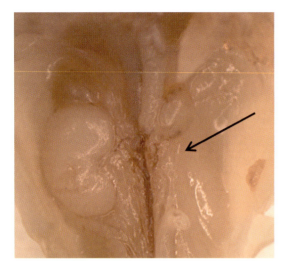

Species	Rat
Memo	Absent kidney: Left kidney is absent.
	腎臓欠損：左腎臓が欠損している。

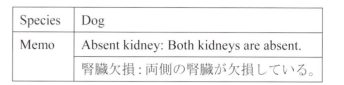

Species	Dog
Memo	Absent kidney: Both kidneys are absent.
	腎臓欠損：両側の腎臓が欠損している。

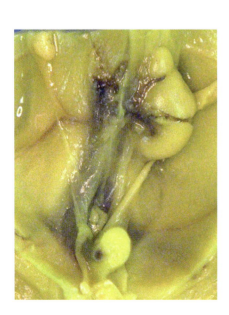

Species	Rat
Memo	Absent kidney (right) with Malpositioned ovary (left, 10386)
	腎臓欠損：右腎臓が欠損している。卵巣位置異常（10386）を伴う。

7-10 Cyst in the kidney　腎臓嚢胞　(10328)

Species	Mouse
Memo	Cyst in the kidney with Distended urinary bladder (10354): Cyst is observed in the left kidney.
	腎臓嚢胞：左腎臓に嚢胞、膀胱拡張（10354）を伴う。

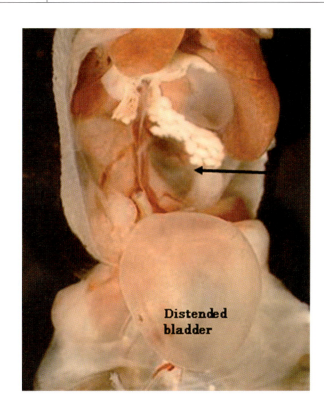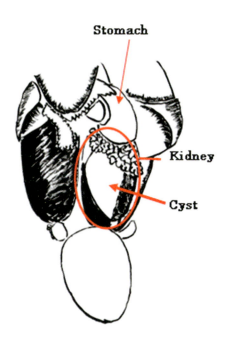

7-11　Large kidney　腎臓大型（化）　(10331)

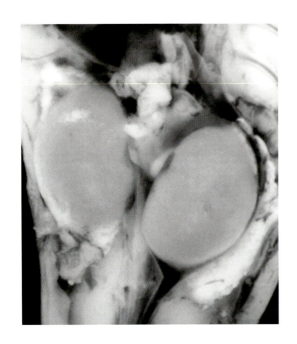

Species	Rabbit
Memo	Large kidney: Both kidneys are large
	腎臓大型（化）：両側の腎臓が大きい。

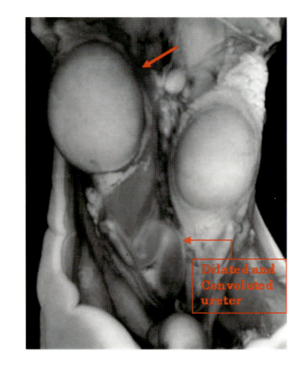

Species	Rabbit
Memo	Large kidney with Dilated ureter (right, 10358) and Convoluted ureter (right, 10357): Right kidney is also called "Hydronephrosis (10334 in Ver. 1)".
	腎臓大型（化）：右腎臓が大型（化）。水腎（旧 10334）であり、尿管拡張（10358）及び尿管蛇行（10357）を伴う。

7-12　Fused kidney　腎臓癒合　(10332)

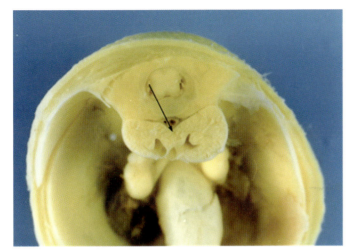

Species	Rat, SD
Memo	Fused kidney: Both kidneys fused.
	腎臓癒合：左右の腎臓が癒合している。

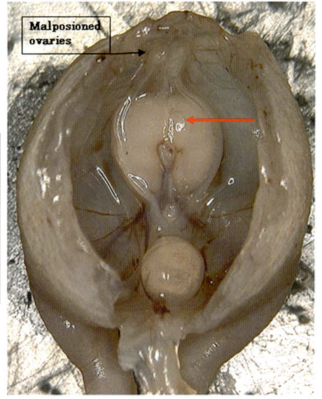

Species	Rat
Memo	Fused kidney with Malpositioned ovary (10386): Both kidneys fused. In human, this is called as "Horseshoe kidney", however this is not a preferred term in the harmonization of terminology in experimental animals.
	腎臓癒合：左右の腎臓（上部）が癒合している。卵巣位置異常（両側、10386）を伴う。
	ヒトでは馬蹄腎（動物ではNon-preferred termであるが）とも言う。

7-12　Continued

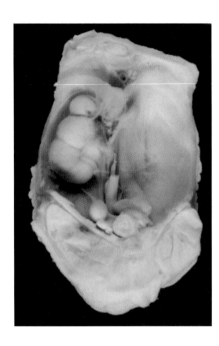

Species	Rat
Memo	Fused kidney with Absent adrenal (left, 10343): Left kidney is transposed to the right-side and fuses with the right kidney.
	腎臓癒合：左腎臓が右側に移動し、癒合している（尿管は 2 本確認できる）。副腎欠損（左、10343）を伴う。

7-13　Misshapen kidney　腎臓形態異常　(10337)

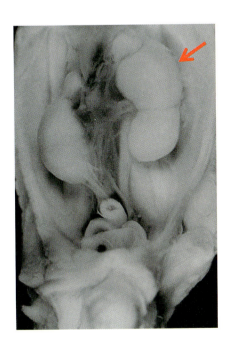

Species	Rat
Memo	Misshapen kidney: The left kidney is large and abnormally shaped. This also can be classified as "Duplicated and Fused kidney", however, it is better to be "Misshapen" because of a single ureter from this large kidney.
	腎臓形態異常：左腎臓が大きく、形が異常。腎臓が過剰で癒合しているとも判断できるが、尿管は1本であり「形態異常」が望ましい。

7-14   Small kidney   腎臓小型(化)   (10339)

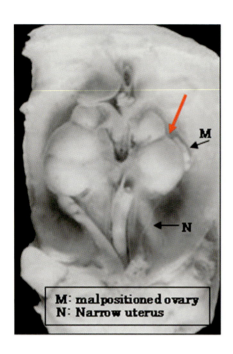

Species	Rat
Memo	Small kidney (left) with Malpositioned ovary (left, 10386) and Narrow uterus (left, New): The left kidney is small.
	腎臓小型(化)：左腎臓が小型。左卵巣位置異常（10386）及び左子宮狭窄（New）を伴う。

7-15 Dilated renal pelvis　腎盂拡張　(10329)

Species	Rat
Memo	Dilated renal pelvis with Dilated ureter (10358): Renal papilla cannot be observed.
	腎盂拡張：腎乳頭が認められない。尿管拡張（10358）を伴う。

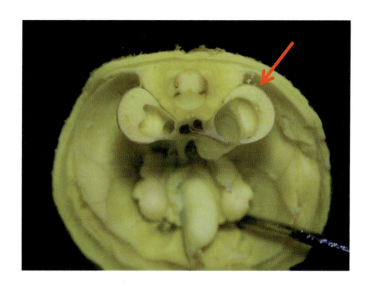
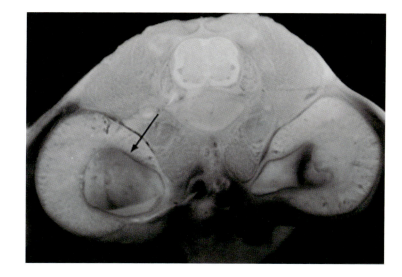

7-16 Absent adrenal 副腎欠損 (10343)

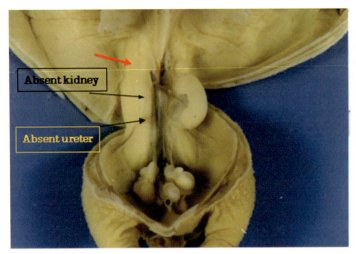

Species	Rat, SD
Memo	Absent adrenal (right) with Absent kidney (right, 10326) and Absent ureter (right, 10356)
	副腎欠損（右）：腎臓の欠損（右 10326）及び尿管欠損（右 10356）を伴う。

7-17 Discolored adrenal 副腎変色 (New)

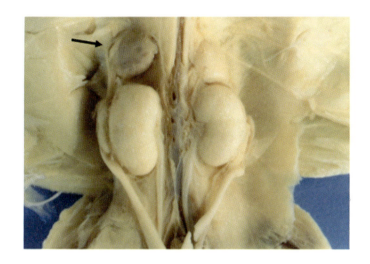

Species	Rat, SD
Memo	Discolored adrenal (right) with Large adrenals (both, 10344)
	副腎変色：右の副腎が変色している。両側の副腎は大型（化）を伴う。

7-18   Large adrenal   副腎大型（化）   (10344)

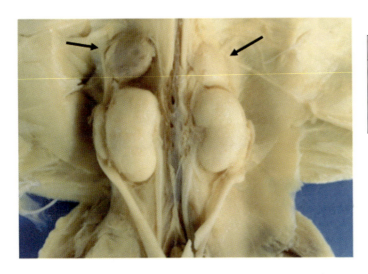

Species	Rat, SD
Memo	Large adrenal (Both) with Discolored adrenal (right, New)
	副腎大型（化）：両側の副腎が大型化している。右副腎は変色（New）を伴う。

7-19 Absent urinary bladder 膀胱欠損 (10352)

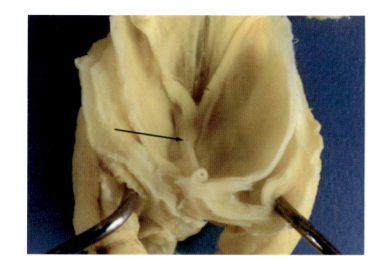

Species	Rat, SD
Memo	Absent urinary bladder, Acystia
	膀胱欠損

7-20 Distended urinary bladder　膀胱拡張　(10354)

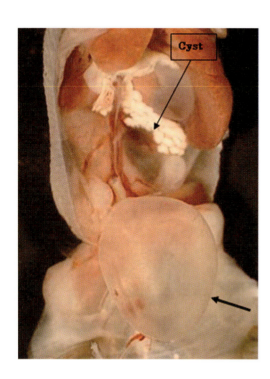

Species	Mouse
Memo	Distended urinary bladder (thick arrow) with Cyst in the left kidney (thin arrow, 10328)
	膀胱拡張（太矢印）：左腎臓嚢胞（細矢印、10328）を伴う。

7-21　Absent ureter　尿管欠損　(10356)

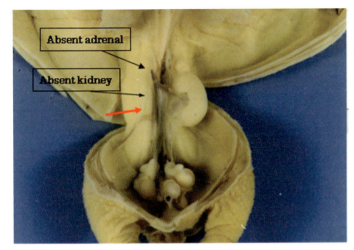

Species	Rat, SD
Memo	Absent ureter (right) with Absent adrenal (right, 10343) and Absent kidney (right, 10326)
	尿管欠損：右腎臓の欠損（10326）に伴い、右尿管が欠損している。副腎欠損（右 10343）を伴う。

7-22　Convoluted ureter　尿管蛇行　(10357)

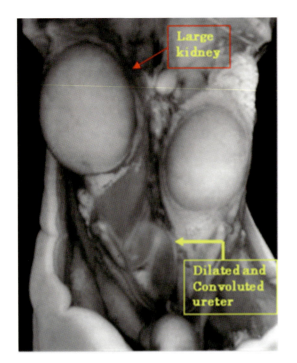

Species	Rabbit
Memo	Convoluted ureter (right) with Large kidney (right, 10331) and Dilated ureter (right, 10358)
	尿管蛇行（右）：右尿管が蛇行している。腎臓大型（化）｛10331、所謂、水腎（旧10334）｝及び尿管拡張（化）（10358）を伴う。

Species	Rat
Memo	Convoluted ureter with Distended ureter (10358)
	尿管蛇行：尿管拡張（10358）を伴う。

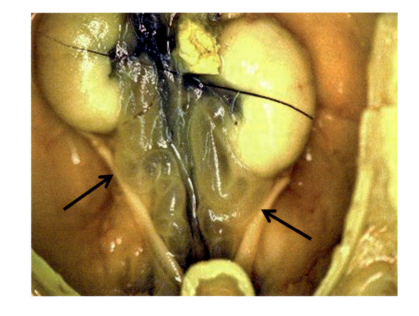

7-23 Dilated ureter　尿管拡張　(10358)

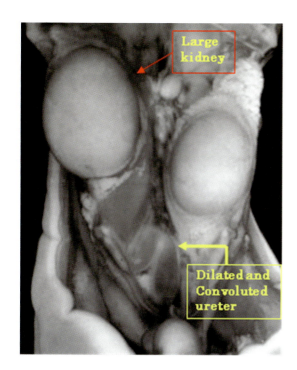

Species	Rabbit
Memo	Dilated ureter (right) with Large kidney (right, 10331) and Convoluted ureter (right, 10357)
	尿管拡張（右）：右尿管が拡張（化）。腎臓大型（化）{10331、所謂、水腎（旧 10334）} 及び尿管蛇行（10357）を伴う。

Species	Rat
Memo	Dilated ureter with Convoluted ureter (10331)
	尿管拡張：尿管蛇行（10331）を伴う。

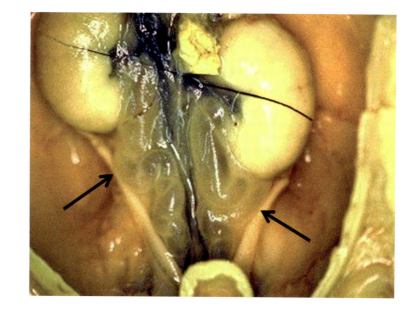

Photographs of Visceral Anomalies

8. Reproductive Organs

8-1 Absent testes　精巣欠損　(10366)

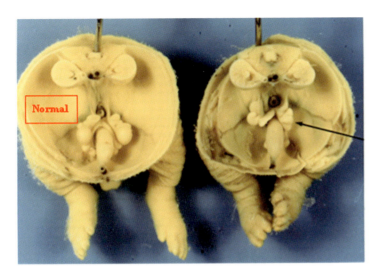

Species	Rat, SD
Memo	Absent testes: Both testes are absent although both epididymides are present.
	精巣欠損：両側の精巣が欠損している。副生殖器（精巣上体）は存在する。

8-2 Malpositioned testis　精巣位置異常　(10369)

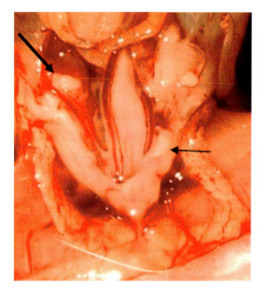

Species	Rabbit
Memo	Malpositioned testis (right): The right testis does not descend to the lower pelvic region.
	精巣位置異常：右精巣が下降していない。

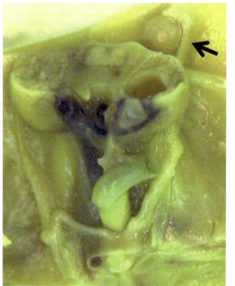

Species	Rat
Memo	Malpositioned testis (left) with Dilated renal pelvis (10329): The left testis does not descend to the lower pelvic region.
	精巣位置異常：左精巣が下降していない。腎盂拡張（10329）を伴う。

8-2 Continued

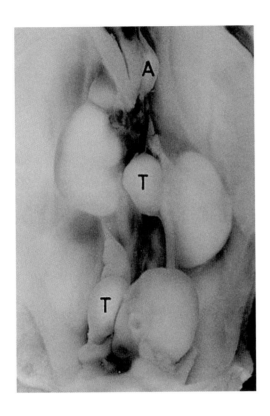

Species	Rat
Memo	Malpositioned testis (left): The left testis does not descend to the lower pelvic region.
	精巣位置異常：左精巣が下降していない。

8-3　Malpositioned ovary　卵巣位置異常　(10386)

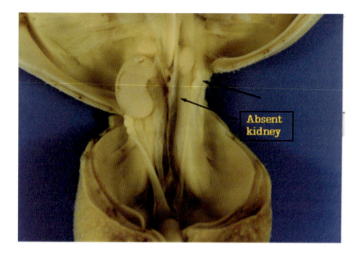

Species	Rat, SD
Memo	Malpositioned ovary (left) with Absent kidney (left, 10326): The left ovary does not descend ventrally in the abdominal cavity.
	卵巣位置異常：左卵巣が上方にズレている。腎臓欠損（左 10326）を伴う。

Species	Rat
Memo	Malpositioned ovary (both side) with Fused kidney (10332): Both ovaries do not descend ventrally in the abdominal cavity.
	卵巣位置異常：両側の卵巣が上方（腎臓の上部）にズレている。腎臓癒合（10332）を伴う。

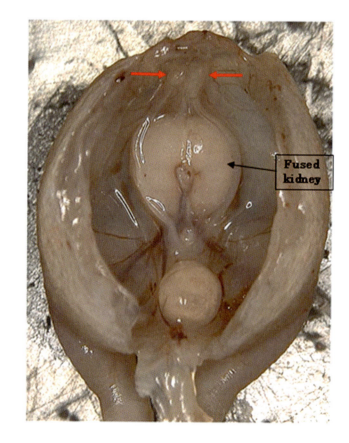

8-3 Continued

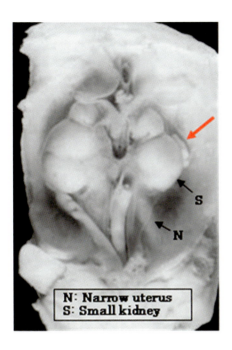

Species	Rat
Memo	Malpositioned ovary (left) with Narrow uterus (left, New) and Small kidney (left, 10339): The left ovary does not descend ventrally in the abdominal cavity.
	卵巣位置異常：左卵巣が腎臓上部にある。腎臓小型（化）（左、10339）及び子宮狭窄（左、New）を伴う。

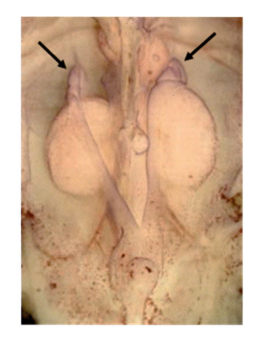

Species	Rat
Memo	Malpositioned ovary: Both ovaries do not descend.
	卵巣位置異常：両側の卵巣が下降していない。

8-4 Narrow uterus 子宮狭窄 (New)

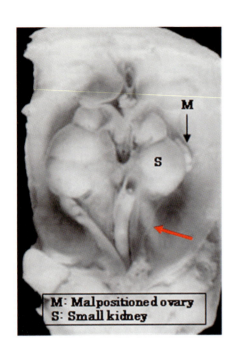

Species	Rat
Memo	Narrow uterus (left) with Malpositioned ovary (left, 10386) and Small kidney (left, 10339): The left uterus horn is generally narrow.
	子宮狭窄（左）：左子宮角が全体に狭窄している。卵巣位置異常（左、10386）及び腎臓小型（化）（左、10339）を伴う。

8-5　**Small uterus**　子宮小型（化）　**(10401)**

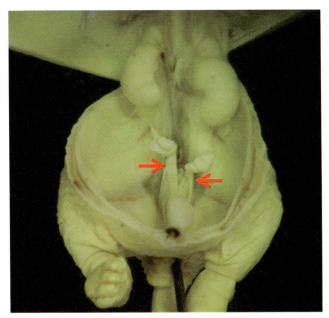

Species	Rat, SD
Memo	Small uterus: Both horns reduced in size, and the position of both ovaries is far from the kidneys.
	子宮小型（化）：両側の子宮角が小さい。卵巣の位置も腎臓から離れている。

8-6 **Absent uterine horn** 子宮角欠損 **(10397)**

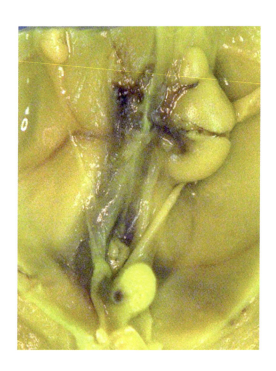

Species	Rat
Memo	Absent uterine horn with Absent kidney (right, 10326): The right uterine horn is rudimentary.
	子宮角欠損：右子宮角が痕跡状である。腎臓欠損（右、10326）を伴う。

Atlas of Developmental Anomalies in Experimental Animals
実験動物発生異常アトラス

Visceral Anomalies
内臓異常

2015 年 5 月 20 日　第 1 刷発行

編集　日本先天異常学会用語委員会
Edited by Project of the Terminology Committee of the Japanese Teratology Society

発行　株式会社 薬事日報社　YAKUJI NIPPO, LTD.
http://www.yakuji.co.jp
本社　東京都千代田区神田和泉町 1
電話　(03) 3862-2141
支社　大阪市中央区道修町 2-1-10
電話　(06) 6203-4191

印刷・製本　昭和情報プロセス株式会社

落丁本・乱丁本はお取り替えいたします。本書の無断複製を禁じます。